GERIATRICS, GERONTOLOGY AND ELDERLY ISSUES

ELDERLY CARE

CURRENT ISSUES AND CHALLENGES

Geriatrics, Gerontology and Elderly Issues

Additional books and e-books in this series can be found on Nova's website under the Series tab.

GERIATRICS, GERONTOLOGY AND ELDERLY ISSUES

ELDERLY CARE

CURRENT ISSUES AND CHALLENGES

SEAN M. ECKSTEIN
EDITOR

nova
Medicine & Health
New York

NOTICE TO THE READER

Library of Congress Cataloging-in-Publication Data

Names: Eckstein, Sean M., editor.
Title: Elderly care : current issues and challenges / Sean M. Eckstein,editor.
Description: New York : Nova Science Publishers, [2020] | Series: Geriatrics, gerontology and elderly issues | Includes bibliographical references and index. | Identifiers: LCCN 2020035215 (print) | LCCN 2020035216 (ebook) | ISBN 9781536184464 (hardcover) | ISBN 9781536185393 (adobe pdf)
Subjects: LCSH: Older people--Services for. | Older people--Care. | Social workers--Training of. Classification: LCC HV1451 .E4683 2020 (print) | LCC HV1451 (ebook) | DDC
362.6--dc23
LC record available at https://lccn.loc.gov/2020035215
LC ebook record available at https://lccn.loc.gov/2020035216

Published by Nova Science Publishers, Inc. † New York

CONTENTS

Preface		**vii**
Chapter 1	Addressing Ethical Issues in the Design of Patient and Caregiver Monitoring Technology in Aged Care Settings *Joan Cahill, Niall O Neill, Sean McLoughlin and Sean Wetherall*	1
Chapter 2	A Review of Assistive Technologies for Activities of Daily Living of Elderly *Nirmalya Thakur and Chia Y. Han*	**61**
Chapter 3	Building a New Vision for Nursing Homes in Lebanon *Marina Gharibian Adra*	**85**
Chapter 4	Elderly Homes and Elderly Care in Lebanon *Ramzi Nasser and Jacqueline Doumit*	**113**
Chapter 5	Care Workers and Quality of Care in Nursing Homes in Canada *Zafar Mehdi and Ramzi Nasser*	**135**

Chapter 6 International Perspectives Regarding Future Development in Nursing Homes: Hong Kong, Japan, and Germany **157**
Shuk Kwan Tang, Mimi M. Y. Tse, Noriko Yamamoto-Mitani and Andrea Budnick

Chapter 7 Older Adults Living in Nursing Homes: Can We Do Something to Enhance Their Happiness and Reduce Their Pain? **169**
Mimi Tse, Shamay NG, Xue Bai, Paul Lee, Raymond Lo and Shuk Kwan Tang

Chapter 8 Desperate Souls: Medicare Home Care Ignores Patient Substance Abuse Assessment and Treatment **177**
William Cabin

Chapter 9 "I Love What I Do" How to Support Home Care Aides in Doing the Work They Love **195**
Sandra S. Butler

Index **209**

PREFACE

Elderly Care: Current Issues and Challenges first presents an analysis of the ethical and societal issues related to the introduction of new patient and care/caregiver monitoring technologies.

A comprehensive review of assisted living technologies aimed at helping elderly people to perform activities of daily living is provided, and associated challenges identified through this review are discussed.

The authors go on to maintain how it is incumbent on the Lebanese government to find ways to invest in economic and social development targeted at providing accessible and high-quality services to its older population to ensure a respectful and independent life.

Socio-demographic changes, social and economic developments, health services and financing relative to the elderly population in Lebanon are discussed in further detail.

Additionally, this compilation investigates the impact of further training of care workers on the quality of care in nursing homes in Canada through a multiple regression analysis technique.

An overview of the aging populations in Hong Kong, Japan, and Germany is presented. The perceptions of nursing homes held by older and middle-aged adults and their expectations of what nursing homes will be like in the future are explored.

Following this, the effects of a non-drug pain management program for older adults in a nursing home environment are assessed.

A review of substance use and abuse coverage in Medicare home health is provided in conjunction with an exploratory study based on interviews of a sample of 26 home care social workers in the New York City metropolitan area.

In closing, the authors discuss the findings of two studies on home care aides in Maine and, from the perspective of the study participants, offer recommendations for improving job conditions.

Chapter 1 - The monitoring and evaluation of patient health and wellbeing, along with the quality of care delivery is critical to patient safety. The aged care sector has faced many scandals about the quality of aged care services. New technologies are being advanced to support patient/resident and care monitoring in acute and aged care settings. The emerging 'surveillance technology' involves a spectrum of intelligence including passive ambient sensors, virtual monitoring, video monitoring and vision systems with different levels of artificial intelligence and machine learning capability. These technologies raise fundamental legal, ethical and societal questions in relation to the meaning of care, privacy and the role of people and technology in delivering care. This chapter presents an analysis of the ethical and societal issues to be addressed in the introduction of new patient and care/caregiver monitoring technologies. The analysis follows several phases of human factors research undertaken by the authors, including an analysis of salient literature around the ethics of monitoring, a meta-analysis of prior aged care studies relevant to the theme of 'monitoring', and a follow up analysis of prior research findings using a human factors and ethics canvas (HFEC). Older people, especially those living with cognitive impairment are a vulnerable group, and their dignity, rights and privacy must be safeguarded. New patient/resident monitoring technology has the potential to enable a safe, person focused, ethical, efficient and accountable care service, if implemented appropriately. Potentially, many of the ethical challenges specified in the HFEC regarding the adoption and deployment of patient/resident monitoring systems (including video and vision systems) have solutions that can be addressed in time and using an integrated human factors and ethics approach. A holistic understanding of the ethical issues surrounding monitoring technologies will help researchers design technologies that will be effective, beneficial and ethical.

Chapter 2 - One of the distinct features of this century has been the population of older adults which has been on a constant rise. Elderly people have several needs and requirements due to physical disabilities, cognitive issues, weakened memory and disorganized behavior, that they face with increasing age. The extent of these limitations also differs according to the varying diversities in elderly, which include age, gender, background, experience, skills, knowledge and so on. These varying needs and challenges with increasing age, limits abilities of older adults to perform Activities of Daily Living (ADLs) in an independent manner. To add to it, the shortage of caregivers creates a looming need for technology-based services for elderly people, to assist them in performing their daily routine tasks to sustain their independent living and active aging. To address these needs, this work consists of making three major contributions in this field. First, it provides a rather comprehensive review of assisted living technologies aimed at helping elderly people to perform ADLs. Second, the work discusses the challenges identified through this review, that currently exist in the context of implementation of assisted living services for elderly care in Smart Homes and Smart Cities. Finally, the work also outlines an approach for implementation, extension and integration of the existing works in this field for development of a much-needed framework that can provide personalized assistance and user-centered behavior interventions to elderly as per their varying and ever-changing needs.

Chapter 3 - Contemporaneously, the ageing population in Lebanon creates a greater need for nursing services which are often provided in residential care facilities. At present, the demand for the services provided by nursing homes significantly exceeds the current supply and, as a result, the need for long-term care is increasing and long-term nursing homes are challenged to recognize and support the culture of their residents at a time when their health needs are increasing, however, quality of life remains less than optimal for many nursing home residents in Lebanon.

Despite the growing awareness of nursing home culture change in Western countries, nursing homes in Lebanon consider care as a process and have a task-oriented approach. The few studies undertaken in Lebanon on nursing home residents addressing their quality of life suggest that there is a need to place an emphasis on restructuring how nursing homes view and deliver care. Developed countries that have started putting into practice the innovative concepts of culture change, aiming at optimal elderly care, can serve as examples for developing countries like Lebanon.

However, for implementing culture change in nursing homes in Lebanon, several challenges exist; the most prominent ones being political/financial instabilities and lack of human resources: added to this is the negative attitudes of the society towards aging.

Irrespective of the existing barriers, there is an urgent need for improving the quality of life of nursing home residents in Lebanon through promoting awareness of culture change principles, and the dissemination of several models of culture change. Research in this field should be undertaken in order to provide an empirical base to guide managers and policy makers in designing appropriate policies.

It is incumbent on the Lebanese Government to find ways to invest in economic and social development targeted at providing accessible and high-quality services to its older population and ensure a respectful and independent life to the older residents.

Chapter 4 - Lebanon is an Arabic speaking country located further east of the Mediterranean Sea. Elderly in Lebanon has reached 11.1% of the population 6.85 million. The Lebanese population demographics have changed over the two decades with immigration of the young to outside the country and consequently older age population has greatly burdened the health care system. Little is known about elderly homes and services provided for the elderly residing in these Lebanese long term care institutions. While the country brandishes itself as leading in health and medical services in the Middle East region, there is still a shortage of health care providers/professionals who are specialized in geriatrics. Even with the very aging population and the growing number of long term care institutions, elderly homes (mostly private) face challenges in support facilities, standard accreditation, professional staffing, oversight to its health services, management, human resources, accreditation, nutritional status and infrastructure capacities. This study/chapter will report the status of elderly homes in Lebanon, including socio-demographic changes, social and economic developments, health services and financing. Lebanon like other developing countries is in need to improve standards, practices and policies, and to enforce their implementations in order to improve the quality of life among elderly home dwellers. There is also a need to ensure the availability of health and social services for older persons and promote their continuing participation in social and productive life. The chapter will provide further discussions and recommendations in the health sector for elderly home dwellers in Lebanon.

Chapter 5 - The Canadian population is rapidly ageing and there is a shortage of skilled care workers such as nurses, elder carers and care assistants in Canadian nursing homes. Care services offer older people in long-term care settings, health, psychological and social support. The advancements in health care knowledge and changing health care environment, make demands on care workers to stay abreast of their knowledge and skills to meet the changing needs of care services in home care settings and residential care facilities. Although there are mandatory and volunteer continuing training programs in long-term care sectors in Canada, the effects of further training of care workers on their career advancement, work situation and quality of care in healthcare and long-term care sector were unclear. The purpose of this chapter is to examine the impact of continuing training of nursing staff in Canadian nursing homes and its association with the quality of care of nursing home residents. Based on theoretical premises of "Lifelong Learning Theory" it is assumed that lifelong learning (further training) of care workers in health care and long-term care is likely to have positive effects on professional development, work situation and quality of patient care. The sample of this study is care workers (nurses, elder carers and care assistants) working in healthcare sector in hospitals, home care settings and long-term nursing homes. This includes care workers; nurses (n = 947), elder carers (n = 493) and care assistants (n = 1140). Data were obtained from the latest Canadian National

Survey of Work and Health of Nurses (2005). The study investigated the impact of further training of care workers quality of care in nursing homes in Canada through a multiple regression analysis technique performed on the data. It was found from this study that further training of nurses has significant and positive association with career mobility of the care workers and quality of care of nursing home residents.

Chapter 6 - The services and care delivered to older adults is often a concern of the community and policy makers. Populations worldwide are aging rapidly and life expectancies are growing. The demand for elderly services to provide support and care to older adults in the community is growing, as is the demand for nursing homes. Governments and societies have to plan for adequate facilities and manpower to provide quality care to their populations. The opinions of the aging population regarding nursing homes should also be taken into consideration. For future planning, the perspectives of middle-aged adults should also be included. They are the older adults and service users of the future. In this chapter, an overview of the aging populations in Hong Kong, Japan, and Germany are presented. The perceptions of nursing homes held by older and middle-aged adults, and their expectations of what nursing homes will be like in the future are explored.

Chapter 7 - Pain is common in older adults, and can lead to various physical and psychological issues. Pain and pain-related situations among elderly people living in nursing homes are even more serious. In this chapter, the authors report the effects of pain situations and a non-drug pain management program for older adults in a nursing home environment.

Chapter 8 - There is extensive literature on the significance of substance use, misuse, and abuse among the elderly in the United States. A literature review indicates no studies on the nature, significance, or impacts of the lack of substance use and abuse coverage in Medicare home health. This chapter presents background on the topic and an initial, exploratory study to address the literature gap, based on interviews of a convenience sample of 26 home care social workers between January 2013 and May 2014 in the New York City metropolitan area. Results indicate social workers believe substance use and abuse occurs frequently among Medicare home health patients;

substance use and abuse is not assessed and treated professionally in Medicare home health; the lack of coverage in Medicare home health results in exacerbation of existing patient physical and mental health conditions, which, in turn, worsen substance use and abuse conditions; the homebound requirement and lack of coverage of transportation and personal care assistants limits home care patients ability to obtain outpatient substance use and abuse treatment; and lack of home-based assessment and treatment contributes to increased home care readmissions, re-hospitalizations, and increased caregiver burden.

Chapter 9 - As our population ages and older adults needing assistance increasingly prefer to say in their homes, the demand for home care aides (HCAs) is growing dramatically. Currently demand for these valuable workers far outweighs supply. It is imperative that we improve job conditions in order to maintain current workers and attract new ones. This chapter will review findings from two studies concerning HCAs in the rural state of Maine. The first, a mixed-method, longitudinal inquiry (n = 261), carried out from 2008 to 2010, examined factors contributing to job turnover for HCAs. Findings indicated that many workers left their home care jobs despite loving the work and feeling very committed to their clients; more than one third of the sample (n = 90) terminated over the 18 months of data collection. Low compensation, lack of benefits, irregular hours, and worker burnout contributed to turnover decisions according to study participants. A more recent in-depth qualitative study examined the structural and psychological components of the HCA job that influence a worker's feeling of empowerment. This inquiry (n = 8; 2018) revealed the deep connections research participants felt with their work and their clients, while simultaneously struggling with challenges such as poor wages, uneven support from agencies, minimal training, and not being adequately valued in the larger health care team. This chapter discusses the findings from both these studies and, from the perspective of the study participants, offer recommendations for improving job conditions so as to make recruitment of new workers easier and retention of current workers more likely.

In: Elderly Care
Editor: Sean M. Eckstein

ISBN: 978-1-53618-446-4

Chapter 1

ADDRESSING ETHICAL ISSUES IN THE DESIGN OF PATIENT AND CAREGIVER MONITORING TECHNOLOGY IN AGED CARE SETTINGS

Joan Cahill[1,*], Niall O Neill[2], Sean McLoughlin[2] and Sean Wetherall[2]

[1]School of Psychology, Trinity College Dublin, Dublin, Ireland
[2]Oneview Healthcare, Dublin, Ireland

ABSTRACT

The monitoring and evaluation of patient health and wellbeing, along with the quality of care delivery is critical to patient safety. The aged care sector has faced many scandals about the quality of aged care services. New technologies are being advanced to support patient/resident and care monitoring in acute and aged care settings. The emerging 'surveillance technology' involves a spectrum of intelligence including passive ambient

* Corresponding Author's Email: cahilljo@tcd.ie.

sensors, virtual monitoring, video monitoring and vision systems with different levels of artificial intelligence and machine learning capability. These technologies raise fundamental legal, ethical and societal questions in relation to the meaning of care, privacy and the role of people and technology in delivering care. This chapter presents an analysis of the ethical and societal issues to be addressed in the introduction of new patient and care/caregiver monitoring technologies. The analysis follows several phases of human factors research undertaken by the authors, including an analysis of salient literature around the ethics of monitoring, a meta-analysis of prior aged care studies relevant to the theme of 'monitoring', and a follow up analysis of prior research findings using a human factors and ethics canvas (HFEC). Older people, especially those living with cognitive impairment are a vulnerable group, and their dignity, rights and privacy must be safeguarded. New patient/resident monitoring technology has the potential to enable a safe, person focused, ethical, efficient and accountable care service, if implemented appropriately. Potentially, many of the ethical challenges specified in the HFEC regarding the adoption and deployment of patient/resident monitoring systems (including video and vision systems) have solutions that can be addressed in time and using an integrated human factors and ethics approach. A holistic understanding of the ethical issues surrounding monitoring technologies will help researchers design technologies that will be effective, beneficial and ethical.

Keywords: patient monitoring, care quality, safety/risk assessment, patient safety, assisted living, residential care, surveillance technology, video monitoring, vision systems, ethics, acceptability, human factors

INTRODUCTION

Background

Monitoring is typically defined in relation to observing or maintaining regular surveillance over a person or something for a prescribed time period. Usually, this involves some form of 'sensing' such as looking and listening. In healthcare, 'sensing' pertains to patient assessment and care delivery and follows a predefined reporting structure in line with clinical assessment criteria and allied care processes.

Older adults in aged care reflect a spectrum of needs and abilities. Typically, the nature and level of monitoring reflects (1) the ability/needs of the person and (2) the setting type. Persons domicle in assisted living enviroments experience less direct montioring than those in palliative care or acute care settings.

The monitoring and evaluation of patient health and wellbeing, along with the quality of care delivery is critical to patient safety. Recent studies indicate that approximately 10% of hospital admissions are associated with an adverse event (Rafter et al., 2014). This can include patient falls, medication errors, hospital acquired infections (HAPS) and pressure sores. The rate of clinical incidences resulting in patient harm is higher for older persons and those with disability and cognitive impairment (State Claims Agency, 2015).

The aged care sector has faced many scandals about the quality of aged care services. Care providers must provide assurances that care is of an appropriate standard and in line with care standards. Older people, especially those living with cognitive impairment are a vulnerable group. In care settings, family members/friends play an important role in relation to monitoring the quality of care and advocating on behalf of the resident/patient (relational autonomy). Often family members fill care gaps/breaches. These protections are not in place for persons with limited social ties/family participation. Given this, such persons are potentially more at risk in relation to poor quality care and neglect.

Research Problem

New technologies are being advanced to support patient/resident and care monitoring in acute care (Zielazinski, 2019) and aged care settings (Adelman, 2002). The emerging 'surveillance technology' involves a spectrum of intelligence including passive ambient sensors, virtual monitoring, video monitoring and vision systems with different levels of artificial intelligence and machine learning capability. The ethics of surveillance been a controversial issue for some time (Social Care Instiute for Excellence, 2014; Mortenson et al., 2013). New patient and caregiver monitoring technologies (and specifically video monitoring technologies linked to operational intelligence) raise fundamental legal, ethical and societal questions in relation to privacy, the meaning of care and the role of people and technology in delivering care. This includes questions about the importance of the human role in care, the role of the resident/patient in healthcare decision making (and family involvement), and what value we place on protecting the personal sphere. Does this new monitoring technology enhances patient experience and safety, or is it a harmful substitute for human/social interaction? Currently, there is a paucity of research evidence as to (1) issues pertaining to ethics, (2) user acceptability and (3) a suitable implementation approach.

Chapter Overview

This chapter presents an analysis of the ethical and societal issues to be addressed with the introduction of new patient and care/caregiver monitoring technologies. The analysis follows from the integration of several phases of human factors research undertaken by the authors. This includes an analysis of salient literature around the ethics of monitoring (phase 1), a meta-analysis of prior aged care studies releant to the theme of 'monitoring' (phase 2), and a follow up analysis of prior research findings using a human factors and ethics canvas (phase 3). In so doing, it analyses these technologies from the perspective of the lived experience, goals and needs of relevant stakeholders, and potential adoption enablers and barriers (Cahill et al., 2018; Cahill et al., 2019). Further, it discusses the importance of locating these new technologies from a 'socio-technical systems design' approach. Specifically, it demonstrates how the 'Systems Engineering Initiative for Patient Safety' (SEIPS) model of work system and patient safety can be used as a framework for understanding the structures, processes and outcomes in health care and their relationships (Carayon et al., 2015), and by implication the requirements for a proposed care monitoring technology addressing diverse stakeholder perspectives.

The chapter opens with a short introduction to healthcare and associated monitoring concepts. Following this, an overview of surveillance and its application in healthcare and associated ethical issues is presented. A summary of underlying human factors and ethical theory is then presented. This theory is relevant to the conceptual framework used in this study, the specific analysis of the ethical implications of new monitoring technologies, and the definition of an ethically responsible monitoring solution. The research question and allied methodology is then presented. Following this, the results of the first two phases of research are detailed. The results of the third phase of research are then presented. This involves an analysis of new patient and care monitoring technology using the Human Factors & Ethics Canvas as advanced by Cahill (2019). The human factors/ethics problem and solution recommendations are then discussed and some conclusions drawn.

Introduction to Healthcare and Monitoring in Healthcare

Health systems include "all organizations, institutions and resources "whose primary purpose is to promote, restore and/or maintain health" (WHO, 2013). The primary stakeholder is the patient. Other key stakeholders include caregivers and clinicians, family members and care facility owners.

Care is delivered across a range of settings. As defined by WHO (2019), acute care or secondary healthcare services are "responsive to life-threatening emergencies, acute exacerbation of chronic illnesses and many routine health problems that nevertheless require prompt action". Aged care settings are diverse and include care in the home, community monitoring, acute care services, post-acute care services, assistive living communities/residential care and palliative care. The type of care provided after a period of acute care is known as post-acute care. Care in the home can include formal and informal care. Older adults living at home/in the community often attend community day services. Such services span the biopsychosocial dimensions of health and wellbeing. Assisted living/residential care settings are defined as group living environments for adults with disabilities and/or older adults who require assistance with at least one activity of daily living. In many cases, older adults may have some level of cognitive and functional decline. Assisted living facilities follow a social model of care (i.e., beyond bio-medical). Importantly, it is expected that residents live in an environment that resembles home and enables personal autonomy and social connection (Cahill et al., 2017).

Traditionally, health monitoring is performed by the care team and recorded on paper. This has relied on nurse/care giver observations and the idea of putting 'eyes' on the person (i.e., following the concept of observation). In all settings, monitoring follows the requirements of care assessment and planning and adheres to compliance/regulatory standards. In acute/hospital settings, monitoring mostly addresses the patient's physical health and spans treatment and aftercare processes. Most often, biomarkers are tracked. Care monitoring in assisted living and residential care settings, focuses on the holistic wellbeing of the person/resident and not only on physical health.

Across all settings, certain physical locations are associated with concepts of privacy. As such, there is a clear distinction between a patient/resident's room (i.e., private space) and public and/or social spaces which is either accessible to others and/or shared with others (i.e., other patients/residents, visitors and care staff). In aged care environments, there is a strong focus on creating and maintaining a 'home like' environment. The concept of 'home' is important as residents are mostly domicile for long term time periods (Cahill et al., 2017, Cahill et al., 2018; Cahill et al., 2019).

Patient experience spans the emotional, social and physical experience of the patient, while in hospital. It reflects the 'occurrences and events that happen independently and collectively across the continuum of care' (Wolf et al., 2014). A positive patient experience is underpinned by concepts of dignity and respect for patients. Further, it involves the treatment of patients and their families as 'partners in care' and associated clinical decision making (Hewitson, Skew, Graham, Jenkinson & Coulter, 2014).

Patient engagement is defined as a patient's own engagement in their health, their care, and their treatment (Picker Institute, 2008; National Health Service, 2011).

The Institute of Medicine define patient safety as 'the prevention of harm to patients' (Aspden et al., 2004). Emphasis is placed on the system of care delivery that (1) prevents errors; (2) learns from the errors that do occur and (3) is built on a culture of safety that involves the participation of health care professionals, organizations, and patients (Aspden et al., 2004).

INTRODUCTION TO SURVEILLANCE AND ETHICAL ISSUES PERTAINING TO SURVEILLANCE IN HEALTHCARE

In the 18th century, Bentham introduced a novel system of institutional surveillance associated with the concept of the 'panopticon' (Jennings, 2012). The panopticon enabled inmates in a prison to be observed by a single security guard without the inmates knowing whether they are being watched. The design concept is premised on the idea that if inmates do not know when they are being watched, they will be motivated to act as though they are being continuously watched. As defined by Foucault (1975), this type of surveillance should be interpreted as a form of punishment. In this case, fear is used to constrain human autonomy (Foucault, 1975).

The use of technology for surveillance has become increasingly pervasive in health and care settings (Desai, 2009; Woolrych et al., 2013). While there is a long history of surveillance of those living in institutional settings, the availability and range of new technologies now provides more options for care providers. Video surveillance (also called closed-circuit television (CCTV)) is already widely used in public and common areas of hospitals and residential care settings (Kohl, 2002). However, these technologies are now being extended to private spaces (i.e., patient/resident rooms). New surveillance technologies are being introduced to enhance patient safety, to reduce staff workload and to improve efficiency (and thereby reduce costs). Overall, the objective is to use technology to provide a holistic picture of the state of person, their environment, and the quality of care delivery (Cahill et al., 2019) – albeit in a cost-effective and legal manner.

Such technologies have been advanced to address the requirements of different stakeholder groups (for example, patients/residents, care staff and family) and specific care problems (for example, caregiver workload, potential for neglect of older adults, falls prediction etc). Surveillance technology provides an alternative to traditional safety/risk mitigation approaches implemented in aged care settings. For example, it can replace the use of restraints and locked doors (traditionally used for older adults at risk of falls and/or wandering). It is also an alternative to 'sitters' – including both physical sitters and virtual sitters, which are often used for persons necessitating continuous monitoring. This technology is also being used to provide protections in relation to preventing elder abuse and neglect. As such, it bolsters and in many cases, replaces existing risk management and safety processes for high risk and/or high dependency patients/residents.

The beneficent uses of technology have a way of being co-opted for other purposes (Brobst, 2018). In relation to privacy, care organisations have privacy obligations to residents and employees and cannot have 'hidden-camera situations' in private areas. The introduction of new data protection legislation in Europe in 2016 has raised new questions concerning the use of health data and privacy issues. General Data Protection Regulation (GDPR) treats health data as a 'special category' of personal data which is considered to be sensitive by its nature (EU, 2020). Further, there are concerns in relation to the potention reduction in social interaction arising from replacing human observation/interaction with machine observation/ interaction. Potentially, a reduction in person to person interaction between caregivers and patients/residents may have negative results on an older adults wellbeing.

Design/technology teams exercise choice in relation to what is valued and advancing technology that improves the human condition. Overall, the objective is to provides benefit and not harm. In line with evidenced based approaches in healthcare (Miake-Lye et al., 2016), evidence is required to justify an appropriate balance between benefit and harm, and a suitable implementation approach. In this case, to provide ethical justification for patient/care montioring technology, the potential benefit in relation to patient experience/safety through monitoring must be balanced with the potential harm of monitoring. Design/technology teams must carefully consider the human dimensions of this technology, its purpose and intended use, implications in relation to human identity and rights, social and care implications and broader societal implications. Overall, there needs to be clear indicators of the benefits including psychosocial benefits (i.e., wellbeing, social participation, autonomy and perceived safety).

Of course, video montioring needs to be situated in the context of recent trends which are changing concepts of care and privacy. The introduction of video cameras follows from several relevant healthcare technology trends. This includes the quantified self, patient self-management of health (for example, self management in relation to renal or diabetes care) and smart home technologies (i.e., passive sensors installed in an older adults home that allow for passive monitoring of health and activity). It also follows from new trends in relation to data intelligence such as real time event orchestration and personalised medicine. These are discussed in more detail in later sections.

Theoretical Frameworks: Human Factors, Human Factors in Healthcare and Ethics

Human Factors

As defined in ISO 6385, the discipline of human factors (HF) refers to 'the practice of designing products, systems, or processes to take proper account of the interaction between them and the people who use them' (2016). Human factors research applies theory, principles, data and methods to design to optimize human well-being and overall system performance. Importantly, it addresses the functions and benefit of technology from the perspective of all relevant stakeholders. Critically, the human factors approach follows a 'socio-technical systems design' perspective. This is an approach to organizational work design that recognizes the interaction between people/behavior, technology/tools, work processes, workplace environments and work culture (Baxter & Sommerville, 2011). As such, the introduction of new technology is conceived as one of many behavior and organizational change interventions. By implication, we must situate any patient monitoring technology in the context of the design of a broader socio-technical system – including caregiver training, safety culture, the design of care and assessment processes and so forth. Another key aspect of the 'human factors approach' is the importance it places on the person. In the context of aged care, this includes the older adult and the care and clinical teams that support them. A critical tenet in HF is the idea that work processes and the design of the overall care system should be designed so that the person (i.e., the caregiver and/or the clinical team) is set-up for success.

Work Design and Patient Safety in Healthcare

Healthcare is now adapting human factors principles and concepts, and specifically the human factors concept of 'person-centered sociotechnical system' (Waterson, 2009). This is evidenced by the application of the Systems Engineering Initiative for Patient Safety {SEIPS 1.0 and SEIPS 2.0} (Carayon et al., 2006). As stated in the SEIPS model, the structure of an organization (or, more generally, the work system) affects how safely care is provided (i.e., the process). Further, the means of caring for and managing the patient (i.e., the process) affects how safe the patient is (i.e., the outcome). As defined in the model, technology designers must consider the relationship between outcomes for patients, service providers/care givers and care organization (i.e., interrelated outcomes). By implication, new monitoring technology needs to deliver benefits for different stakeholders. Any proposed system must be jointly optimized for patients and caregivers alike.

Ethics, Digital Ethics and Data Ethics

Overall, ethics concerns the moral principles that govern a person's behavior or how an activity is conducted. A key distinction in ethics is the distinction between that which is unethical and that which is undesirable. Primarily, moral principles apply to a person. However, moral code can also be ascribed to the behavior of automated or intelligent systems (A/IS).

'Digital ethics' or information ethics deals with the impact of digital Information and Communication Technologies (ICT) on our societies and the environment at large (Capurro, 2019). As defined 'it addresses the ethical implications of things which may not yet exist, or things which may have impacts we cannot predict' (Capurro, 2019).

Data ethics is defined as 'A branch of ethics that evaluates data practices with the potential to adversely impact on people and society – in data collection, sharing and use' (ODI, 2018).

Rights

Rights are the fundamental normative rules concerning what a person is entitled to. Philosophers distinguish between negative and positive rights. A positive right is a right to be subjected to an action or another person or group. A negative right is a right not to be subjected to an action of another person or group. The Universal Declaration of human rights (1948) enshrines all persons with human rights. This includes rights pertaining to dignity (Article 1), autonomy (Article 3), privacy (Article 12), and safety (Article 29).

Charters of rights for older adults living in care homes have been advanced both generally (European Commission, 2010) and in the memory care context (Alzheimer's Society of Ireland, 2013). The charters highlight certain principles that should be considered in relation to the introduction of new monitoring technologies. For example, patient/resident consent in relation to the use of specific technologies/sensors and associated information captured, and the protection of the personal sphere. In addition, the above charters recognize that autonomy in navigating both privacy and social interaction are essential to human well-being and the fulfilment of human potential.

Application of Moral Theory in Relation to New Technology Design

Many ethical theories have been used to examine the ethical issues pertaining to new technologies. Two main classical theories – namely, Consequentialism and Deontology are often used in relation to the analysis of technology innovation from the perspective of potential benefit versus harm. Consequentialism is the view that normative properties depend only on consequences (Scheffler, 1988). In this theory, the consequences of one's behavior/action are the ultimate basis for any judgment about the rightness or wrongness of that behavior/action. In contradistinction, Deontologists argue that the morality of a given behavior/action should be based on whether that action itself is right or wrong under a series of rules, rather than based on the consequences of the action (Thomas, 2015). As highlighted by Moor (1999), a combination of two is required.

Principlism is an approach to the examination of moral dilemmas based upon the application of certain ethical principles. Principlism provides for a way of 'ethical reasoning that is based on a core set of ethical principles that are not limited by any particular case or by specific theoretical constraints' (Beever & Brightman, 2015).

Exploring Ethical Issus and Ethics Canvas

Ethics issues are now being formally explored in healthcare projects. Several new tools have emerged in relation to examining ethical issues pertaining to new technologies. The 'Human Factors & Ethics Canvas (HFEC)' introduced by Cahill (2019) provides a bridge to integrating HF and ethics issues. The objective of the HFEC is to create an evidence map in relation to the specification of an ethically responsible technology solution, that properly addresses human and ethical issues. The ethics canvas reflects an integration of ethics and HF methods, particularly around the collection of evidence using stakeholder evaluation methods (Cousins et al., 2013; Wenger 1998). Specifically, the ethics canvas makes use of the data obtained from literature review and stakeholder evaluation methods (Cahill, 2019). The output of this analysis is used to provide evidence to justify an appropriate implementation of the proposed technology.

METHODS

Introduction

The objective of this study is to understand the ethical and societal issues relating to the future implementation of monitoring technology in diverse aged care environments. This study forms part of a broader human factors project contributing to the development of ambient assistive living (AAL) technologies in aged care and acute care environments. The overall methodology involves building an evidence map (Miake-Lye et al., 2016) in relation to human factors and ethical issues pertaining to new video monitoring technologies.

The research reported on this chapter concerns the first part of a two-part research study. In the first part of this study, no specific stakeholder research was undertaken in relation to the specification of stakeholder requirements for video monitoring technology and its implementation in a clinical context. Rather, inferences are made following the analysis of prior HF studies concerning the application of passive monitoring technologies/AAL technologies in aged care settings (Cahill et al., 2019; 2018), and the analysis of existing literature on the subject (i.e., Part 1 research). As such, Part 1 research is used to scope the preliminary issues pertaining to technology fit and acceptability, and to define the high-level directions for this technology. Following from this, a full acceptability study will be undertaken involving stakeholder participation in relation to requirements specification and clinical implementation (i.e., Part 2 research).

Research Question

The research question is framed in relation to technology acceptability and ethics and is defined as follows: What are the ethical and societal issues pertaining to the implementation of video monitoring technology in aged care settings. This can be broken down into a series of sub-questions:

1. What type of monitoring/sensing is acceptable to different stakeholders (i.e., patients/residents, staff and families)?
2. How should designers and developers of this technology deal with the potential negative consequences/impacts of this technology, in the design stage?
3. How should this technology be implemented in a care setting, to address issues relating to ethics and acceptability for different stakeholders?

Methods: Part 1 Research

As indicated in Table 1, Part 1 research has involved three phases of research. First a review of the literature pertaining to new technology trends in healthcare, the introduction of video monitoring in healthcare and specific ethical issues pertaining to video monitoring was undertaken.

Relevant prior aged care studies undertaken by the authors, in relation to the application of passive monitoring technology in residential settings were then analyzed. This includes themes pertaining to (1) technology and attitudes, (2) potential benefits/harm and (3) implementation in a care context. It should be noted that the assisted living human factors studies focused on passive monitoring and not video monitoring technologies. However, an analysis of stakeholder attitudes to passive monitoring technology yields insights relevant to more active monitoring technologies such as video monitoring and vision technologies. The third phase of research involves the analysis of the two preceding studies in relation application of a 'human factors and ethics canvas' as developed by Cahill (2019). Table 1 below provides a summary of the different research phases.

Table 1. Part 1 Research: breakdown of research phases

Part	Phase	Description	#	Overview of Research	Status
1	1	Literature review	1.1	Review of available literature on emerging technology trends in healthcare – journal articles, grey literature	Complete
			1.2	Video monitoring in healthcare	Complete
			1.3	Meta-analysis of lit pertaining to ethics and patient/care monitoring (monitoring including video monitoring) – mostly prior systematic lit reviews	Complete
	2	Meta-analysis of prior studies – assisted living – monitoring and ethical issues (not specific to video)			Complete
	3	Analysis of research using HF and Ethics Canvas			Complete
2	1	Prototype Development			To Do
	2	Simulation & Participatory Design/Evaluation			To Do
	3	Implementation & Evaluation			To Do

Human Factors and Ethics Canvas

The objective of the human factors and ethics canvas (HFEC) is to create an evidence map in relation to the specification of an ethically responsible technology solution, that properly addresses human and ethical issues (Cahill, 2019). The HFEC allows non-ethicists such as Designers, Human Factors Researchers, Engineers, and Computer Scientists to assess ethical issues pertaining to the emerging technology product. As defined by Cahill (2019), the HFEC involves seven stages. Stage 1 is all about framing the problem. Stage 2 involves understanding how the technology fits to the problem, defining stakeholder goals and needs and the specification of expected benefits for different stakeholders. This is followed by several deep dives. These are: benefits, outcomes and impact (stage 3), personae and scenario (stage 4), data ethics (stage 5) and implementation (stage 6). The final stage (stage 7) presents the outcomes of the preceding analysis.

In line with stakeholder evaluation approaches, the canvas can be evaluated using the 'community of practice' (i.e., comprising internal and external stakeholders). At a minimum, core internal stakeholders/core team members (including an ethicist {if available}, the HF lead, the design lead and the product owner/manager) are involved in completing the canvas.

In this case, as the first part of this study did not involve specific field research around video monitoring, the ethics canvas has made use of the data obtained in the literature review and the meta-analysis of prior human factors studies. The HFEC was populated by the lead HF researcher, following the analysis of several team workshop sessions addressing different phases of the HFEC.

RESULTS: HEALTHCARE TECHNOLOGY TRENDS, VIDEO MONITORING & ETHICAL ISSUES

Healthcare Technology Trends (General)

Quantified Self and Self-Monitoring of Health

Advanced in wearables and mobile phone technologies have led to the rise the 'quantified self' movement. New digital devices allowing self-tracking of health and associated parameters (for example, phsysical activity, sleep and diet) are gaining popularity (Adjana, 2017). This 'self-monitoring' approach is changing both how health and health care delivery is managed, and how health related information is stored and shared. Specifically, this technology enables patients to have direct access to their own health information. Further patients can risk assess themselves against predefined clinical criteria and share relevant reporting information with clinicians.

Ambient Assisted Living and Smart Homes/Rooms

Ambient assisted living (AAL) is defined as "the use of information and communication technologies (ICT) in a person's daily living and working environment to enable them to stay active longer, remain socially connected and live independently into old age". This involves the advancement of AAL/Internet of Things (IoT)/sensor-based infrastructures which make use of machine learning technology. These infrastructures connect a range of devices (i.e., TV, tablet, mobile phones etc.), sensors (environmental sensors and biosensors) and actuators as part of an IoT hub.

Currently, a range of sensors/monitoring technology is in use (Cahill et al., 2019). Overall, specific technologies address different dimensions of a person's health, 'lived experience' and care delivery. Health montioring technology is used to montior specific bio markers such as heart rate, insuline levels, blood pressure and so forth. Presence and location sensors are also used. Presence sensors can be combined with other sensors to provide greater awareness as to the resident's state. For example, when combined with a bed or light sensor, it is possible to detect that the person is awake and their mobility level (i.e., moving around the room). Real-time location systems (RTLS) are also used (i.e., tracking resident/staff locations). Biometric identification (RFID tags) monitor who is in the room (for example, staff, visitors and patient/resident). This is used for monitoring staffing/care and patient/resident activity and visitors (safety). Staff members swipe a RFID card when entering a room. The system then knows when they enter and exit each room. This can be used to track how long a person has been visited for. Further, when correlated with other sensors, it can be used to measure the impact of this visit on the resident's wellbeing. In addition to the benefits for the resident, this also provide metrics for the care team that can help them optimize their time and provide better care. In some care faciliites, Global Positioning Systems (GPS) insoles are used for persons at risk of wandering and or falling. This enable safe and free movement. Timely notifications are provided to staff, if a safety risk is detected.

Falls Sensors and Fall Profiles

Several technologies have been developed to address the issues of falls (Cahill, 2019). For example, at night, bed sensors and passive infrared sensor (PIRs) can observe that the resident has left their bed. This information is uised to activate low-level lighting to the bathroom to reduce the risk of a fall. The bathroom PIR would detect that the resident has entered the bathroom. If the bedroom PIR and bed sensor do not pick up that the resident has returned to their bed within a time parameter, then a notification can be provided to caregivers to check if the resident has fallen.

Resident behaviour profile monitoring is a system of non-intrusive room sensors which utilizes the latest in Thermal sensor technology to monitor the individual behaviour of each resident (Cahill et al., 2019). The system continuously monitors the resident's room for all activity. Intelligent algorithms are used to analyse and learn pattern recognition to identify the position of the resident. This enables live monitoring of physical activity, stumbling, falls, temperature changes, toilet visits and sleeping patterns (Cahill et al., 2019). This information is used to identify hazardous hotspots (i.e., a pattern of stumbling or falls), so that remedial actions can be taken. It is also used to identify trends in relation to room visits (including both care teams and family members). This can support analysis in relation to social and care activity. In the case of fall detection, short message service (SMS) alerts are provided to the care team, so that the resident obtains immediate help (Cahill et al., 2019).

Reporting Technologies

Traditionally health monitoring is performed by the care team and recorded on paper. However, with more modern technology, there are different options available. For example, a resident can proceed with a self-assessment and the data is directly sent to the system. This information can also be co-related with information from other passive sensors, to inform resident wellbeing assessments (Cahill et al., 2018, Cahill et al., 2019).

Equally, digital reporting systems for caregivers have been introduced. These provide efficiencies in relation to care reporting and have additional benefits in relation to reporting standardization.

Digital Hospital and Real time Event Orchestration (Acute Care)

In acute care settings, the concept of the digital hospital has been introduced (Williams, 2019). The digital hospital has three inter-related goals: (1) improving patient safety and health outcomes, (2) enabling care co-ordination and (3) improving efficiency. Primarily, this involves real time information integration across healthcare systems and teams. In this framework, data is gathered to make predictions about the state of the patient and/or the patient's care. Care interventions are delivered as required and with the appropriate care staff (i.e., staff with certified training and competency). This intelligence is linked to resource utilization and workforce analytics, which in turn drives safety and efficiency.

Hospital Safety Management System (SMS/Acute Care) and Safety II

Hosptial safety management systems (SMS's) provide a structured management approach to control safety risks for patients and staff (Ocuupational Health and Safety Administration, 2013). In healthcare (as with other sectors such as aviation), safety management practices are now moving from Safety I to Safety II approaches (Hollnagel, 2014). Safety II involves using data from normal operations to build a risk profile of the operation, to anticipate risk, and to manage risk at an operational level (Hollnagel, 2014; Hollnagel, Wears & Braithwaite, 2015). Within a hospital safety/risk management system, it links to proactive and predictive risk management approaches (i.e., preventing care events) and allied care monitoring and reporting practices. This includes routine monitoring and reporting, care asessment and adverse events reporting. Any patient and care service monitoring using video or vision technology would require some level of integration with these wider safety/risk management approaches.

Personalised Medicine (Acute Care)

Personalised medicine 'is a move away from a 'one size fits all' approach to the treatment and care of patients with a particular condition, to one which uses new approaches to better manage patients' health and targets therapies to achieve the best outcomes in the management of a patient's disease or predisposition to disease' (National Health Service, 2019). It is anticipated that progress in the fields of bioinformatics and biostatistics, advanced analytical tools (e.g., machine learning) and Artificial Intelligence (AI) solutions, will enable increased precision in relation to diagnosis and treatment and overall care provision. A key dimension of this highly personalised diagnosis, is the integration of data available from various sources/sensors.

New Video Monitoring Technologies

Video cameras are now being deployed at the point of care (i.e., in patient/resident rooms) for the purpose of monitoring patient/resident health, safety, care quality and staffing. Overall, the idea is to prevent safety/care events and ensure a faster response to incidents when they arise. The grey literature documents specific implementation cases. For example, this includes

- Predictive safety/risk management (i.e., falls prediction and monitoring, tempering with attached life supporting devices and self-harm)
- Monitoring of staff and care delivery (i.e., monitoring staff members presence in the room, monitoring staff hygiene routines [hand washing] and monitoring care activity)
- Security (i.e., monitoring unauthorized access to a patient/resident's room)
- Mapping behavior patterns/behavioral analysis (i.e., anxiety, aggression and self-harm)

Virtual sitter systems are common in US hospitals. Care staff perform remote/virtual monitoring tasks (i.e., watching real time video recording) and can interact with staff members on the ward.

Passive monitoring technologies (AAL), video monitoring and vision technologies are being combined/integrated, to monitor and prevent care events (i.e., falls and medication errors). Some vision systems are also integrated with Artificial Intelligence (AI) and Machine Learning (ML) systems - providing greater levels of intelligence in relation to reporting on the patient state and predicting care events. For example, vision technology (assessing facial features and expressions) can be used to determine who is in the room, if the patient is awake/asleep, the patient's mood (i.e., if happy, sad or stressed) and if the patient is in pain. When combined with AI and ML technologies, video based technology is used to make inferences about the risk of fall, based on real time evalution of the patient's sitting and standing position, movement and gait (Brown, 2015). Some companies are offering intelligent cloud-based systems (i.e., HD IP CCTV solutions) on a subscription basis. For example, the Truelysafe VSaaS solution (2020).

Critically, the implementation of these systems is addressing privacy issues. For example, one industry provider Ouva (2020) have built the vision analytics into the actual camera. This ensures that separate hardware is not required onsite. This is being positioned as a positive move for privacy because now only the meta data (results of the analytics) leaves the device. Others such as Celeno (2020) are using Wi-Fi radar to understand a person's position and movement. Wi-Fi radar is perceived as cruder than vision analytics, but simpler from a privacy perspective.

In Australia, a new pilot of CCTV in care homes is being implemented (Briggs & Slessor, 2019). Camera footage is monitored 24/7 by a third-party contractor in a year-long trial. The proposed technology can detect excessive noise and movement, triggering an alert to a reviewer who can instantly check the footage to see if an incident has occurred.

Ethics and Monitoring

Overall, we can distinguish issues pertaining to ethics, legal issues and social acceptability issues. There is much overlap between ethical and social acceptability issues, and between ethical and legal issues. Any implementation of this technology requires consideration of these interrelated issues.

As noted by Brobst (2018), there is a difference between observing and watching. As such, the intended use and purpose of these technologies must be carefully considered. Following a review of personal health monitoring (PHM) literature, Middlestadt (2018) has identified eight themes describing the ethical implications of this technology. The identified themes include privacy, autonomy, obtrusiveness and visibility, stigma and identity, medicalization, social isolation, delivery of care, and safety and technological need (Middlestadt, 2018).

Niemeijer et al. (2010) have raised concerns in relation to the potential impact of this technology on the service user-carer relationship and the moral issues associated with this. The introduction of future monitoring technology (including video or the use of other sensors) may reduce face to face interaction between residents and caregivers. Arguably, this might change care norms around person centered care and lead to greater social isolation.

Others argue that awareness of surveillance could have some positive impacts on staff behavior (Desai, 2009). As reported by Desai (2009), if patients/residents can adjust to an increased degree of surveillance, this technology might decrease the stigma of human observation.

The proposed technology needs to be situated in the context of the existing regulatory/legal framework. As such, it needs to comply with data protection legislation and existing employee protections.

RESULTS: ASSISTED LIVING AND PASSIVE MONITORING TECHNOLOGIES

Stakeholder Goals, Needs and Challenges

Security, safety, comfort, autonomy, social participation and resident/patient wellbeing are common concerns for residents/patients, their families, care staff and care facility owners. Older adults, family members, caregivers and facility owners experience many different challenges.

However, for all stakeholders, the primary challenge is (1) ensuring care quality/compliance and patient safety while also delivering (2) a positive resident/patient experience, within the context of a sustainable and affordable healthcare delivery models. Both patient/residents and family members have specific concerns in relation to the impact of these technologies on the lived experience of older adults in residential/assisted living care settings. This includes concerns about the potential reduction in social contact and loneliness, and risk in relation to loss of identity and autonomy.

Care givers generally do the job because they find meaning and value in their work. However, the job is perceived as increasing more difficult – with added workload demands and little time to provide direct personal care to residents. Process compliance and resident reporting is closely monitored. In such environments, there is often a conflict between resident reporting and providing direct person care to residents. Given the high costs of care and funding shortages, there is often a scarcity of resources. This has implications for staffing and has implications in relation to care quality. Challenges to professionalism are frequently reported. There is agreement that staff cannot deliver safe and/or quality care with limited time/resources. Further, staff workload and burnout can be considered a potential contributory factor to care events/harm. Although there is widespread acceptance that workload and burnout issues need to be addressed, there are concerns about the suitability of video monitoring technology as a solution. Staff have apprehensions that patient and care monitoring technology might be implemented for the wrong reasons (i.e., to reduce staffing costs as opposed to dealing with fundamental issues concerning care delivery).

Overall, clinicians are interested in using patient monitoring technology to enhance health outcomes for residents. The application of passive monitoring technology to provide feedback about a resident's health state is perceived as a positive step. Issues pertaining to managing patient privacy and dignity are expected to be managed in relation to specific clinical, nurse rounding/observations and care delivery processes. As such, the technology might be defined in the context of these processes.

At an organizational and operational level, issues pertaining to the costs of care, and specifically, cost efficiency in relation to the monitoring of high dependency patients/residents were reported.

Care compliance emerged as significant issue. This includes following and documenting compliance requirements in relation to privacy/GDPR, care events, complaints processes and dealing with employment law and ethical/legal dimensions of monitoring staff. Also, in most care organizations, there is a mix of temporary and permanent staff. This makes it difficult to maintain a consistent care ethos and culture.

Stakeholder Concerns and Acceptability Issues

Participants referred to having control over certain aspects of their room. This includes room temperature, lighting, the opening and closing of windows and doors, the layout of the room/space and the style of furniture. Much of the environment is shared with others (for example, corridors, communal/social spaces, eating areas and outdoor areas). This has implications in terms of privacy and control. Participants reported an expectation that concepts of privacy and control might vary according to the specific physical space: (1) the resident's room (full control to meet own comfort requirements), and (2) communal/social spaces (no expectation of personal control).

The use of passive technology (i.e., passive sensors in beds and activity monitoring sensors) to monitor resident safety, prevent falls and raise alarms was perceived quite positively. Further participants noted that new wander management technology (i.e., door sensors and sensors in the environment), would be acceptable, if this enabled free movement.

Participants liked the idea that from a resident perspective, much of the technology might be happening in the background (i.e., bed sensors and sensors on windows/doors). All participants emphasized the importance of upholding resident rights and dignity. It was agreed that personal and medical information should not be shared with others without a patients/resident's permission.

Issues around stakeholder attitudes to the use of video in care settings is a potential barrier to the deployment of this technology and must be addressed. As highlighted in the literature, patients/residents and their families have concerns about the intended use and purpose of this technology, issues pertaining to intrusion/privacy, how consent is established, how video data is stored and who has access to it, technology misuse (i.e., hacking of video), the impact of technology-mediated care (i.e., video as a substitute for human contact) and potential consequences in relation to patient wellbeing and the potential for social isolation.

It is important to maintain the human element of care. This is characterized by human presence, responsive communication and empathetic communication. Participants in the HF assisted living studies noted that if monitoring is automated, and in person contact mostly initiated by electronic help requests, then this might become quite isolating for residents (Cahill et al., 2019). For example, it might result in situations where residents only receive in-person contact if this is requested.

Issues around acceptability do not end with patients. Other stakeholders such as staff, families and visitors must be considered too. In relation to staff, there are concerns in terms of the intended purpose and use of this technology, potential negative consequences (i.e., reduction in staffing, impact on staff workload), potential negative impact on carer role (i.e., less in person time with patient/delivering care), changes to process design (i.e., briefing and handover, care monitoring, care assessment, adverse event management and investigations) and legal implications. In relation to families, there are concerns around privacy (i.e., recording of family conversations) and the impact on the relationship between the patient/resident and caregiver. At an organizational level, specific legal aspects need to be addressed. For example, clear guidance is required in relation to defining liability in cases where the technology fails to adequately anticipate a care event and/or provide a notification to caregivers if a care event occurs. Further, processes and policies need to be defined in relation to the use of video in adverse event investigations.

Potential Stakeholder Benefits

Patients/residents and family members are more likely to accept and adopt this technology, if the technology delivers benefits that they are genuinely interested in (i.e., if they are intrinsically motivated). Patients/residents and family members are likely to be motivated by benefits such as patient safety (i.e., predicting potential falls), the prevention of harm/abuse, and enabling autonomy (i.e., free movement and avoiding falls). The capture of data about care activity provides safeguards for caregivers too. If a care event happens, then this data can be used to investigate where the blame (if any) lies. Further, this technology can reduce workload for caregivers, and enable time for more person-centered care (for example, including touch, eye contact and social/verbal interaction).

Human Factors and Ethics Canvas (HFEC), Framing The Technology Problem and Proposed Video Montioring Solution

Formulating the Problem

Values and human and ethical issues are built into how we frame the problem (Cahill, 2019). Thus, it is critical to first clarify the specific problem (or set of problems) that the proposed technology is addressing. Once this is understood, the use/application of the proposed technology and associated ethical dimensions can be considered. Video monitoring might be used to solve a specific problem and/or a suite of problems. Thus, we need to be clear on the scope and nature of the problem. In this case, the problem is multi-dimensional and concerns several interrelated issues concerning patient care and safety. Based on the issues identified in the aforementioned research, this includes:

- Consistency of patient care and ensuring care compliance
- Staff workload impacting on quality of patient care
- Care of vulnerable and/or at risk/high dependency patients – requirement for continuous monitoring (impact on health outcomes)
- Patient safety – unacceptable number of preventable events
- Participation of patient/resident and family in care.

Overall, we would argue that the above problems be treated as ‘information management’ problems – and managed in the context of the digital hospital/digital care. This is discussed in more detail below.

Personas and Scenarios

The above problems need to be conceptualized from different stakeholder perspectives. In this way, multiple stakeholder perspectives must be considered both (1) in relation to framing the problem and (2) identifying the solution. In line with human factors methodologies, we can define different personae and scenarios and use these personae and scenarios to analyze ethical issues. Example personae and scenarios are presented in Table 2.

Table 2. Example setting, personae and scenarios

Setting	Nurse/Caregiver Personae	Older Adult Personae	Scenario Description
Home/ community	Caregiver with limited experience and poor language skills (not native language)	Older adult with early stage Dementia but otherwise healthy living in the community	Routine monitoring Sudden and rapid decline in patient health
Acute Care	Newly trained nurse with high workload	Older adult post-surgery with heart condition	Routine monitoring Staff burnout Family express concern about potential for patient neglect
Post-Acute Care (PAC)	Caregiver with limited experience and poor language skills (not native language)	Independent older adult with knee injury/rehabilitation	Routine monitoring Potential for patient fall
Assisted Living/residential care	Staff nurse with extensive experience in residential care/assisted living	Frail older adult, limited mobility, mild dementia	Routine monitoring Clinical Review of Patient Need & Care Plan Abuse of patient by staff member

Ethics Principles and Proposed Solution

Decision making regarding technology need and implementation must start from a principled basis. The above problems (and associated instantiation in relation to specific personae/scenario), must be further analyzed in relation to pertinent ethical principles. Ethical theories and principles can be used to unpack the core ethical issues pertaining to the implementation of new video monitoring technologies.

This research indicates that the following ethical principles should be considered in relation to solution design:

1. The provision of a caring and compassionate service
2. Enabling equal access to care and consistency of care

3. Enabling equal opportunities for the best health outcomes for all patients/residents
4. Enabling safe care
   a. Prevent adverse events
   b. Reduce unnecessary adverse events
5. Enabling positive experience for patient/resident
6. Enabling patient self-management of health (where appropriate)
7. Enabling positive experience for caregiver (burnout)
8. Protecting the rights of patients and workers – this includes consent, autonomy, privacy, respect and dignity
9. Social justice as the basic premise for the quality of employment and quality of life
10. Patient/resident and staff monitoring needs to comprehensively address the real needs of people (i.e., diversity) and potential adoption barriers
11. Patient/resident and staff monitoring should support workplace wellness (i.e., management of staff morale, workload and fatigue).

These principles should be used to scope the intended use and solution objectives. In line with these principles, the intended use should be around supporting and protecting the patient/resident (with due consideration to healthcare worker needs). The system should be used to protect the patient/resident from harm. It should also be used to support healthcare workers and not to spy on staff and/or reduce the number of staff. Arguably, it is also ethical to support self-management of care for older adults.

Data Ethics

New surveillance technologies raise many questions pertaining to data ethics. This includes what data is collected, how data is collected, how data is stored, how data is accessed, and by whom is it accessed. It also raises questions regarding how the data is used. This relates to the data models and the specific algorithms used to make predictions/decisions about a patient's/resident's holistic health and allied clinical care processes.

In relation to the issue of what data is collected, there are obvious concerns about intrusion. For example, (1) taking images of faces (i.e., including patients, healthcare workers and visitors), (2) recording certain private activities (i.e., toileting and dressing) and (3) recording private conversations between patients/residents and visitors. There are also concerns about establishing consent for collecting such data. This should depend on establishing voluntary consent from patients. Powers of attorney and advance care directives give relatives and carers' certain decision-making powers in the medical context. However, it is unclear whether these extend to decision-making regarding surveillance. Care providers need to carefully analyze a resident's capacity to provide consent, and the surrounding legal context before making any decisions about CCTV in private rooms (Rozenurgs, 2018). Evidently, the process for this must be clearly defined, and include procedures for a variety of situations. For example, this might include the following contexts:

- Patients/residents who are critically sick and unable to provide consent
- Patients/residents with a disability or serious mental health (MH) issue impacting on their ability to provide consent
- Patients/residents with early cognitive decline (ECD) and/or Dementia which may impact on their ability to give consent.

Processes should also be defined in relation care delivery in the absence of consent. Further, care providers will need to establish consent for the use of video recording in private areas.

In addition to establishing processes for consent, clear policies and procedures should also be established around how surveillance is implemented from a care delivery and staffing perspective. This includes procedures in relation to:

- Access to video data
- How video data is presented to relevant stakeholders
- How video data is used in relation to making decisions about care – for example, how video data is used in clinical assessments
- How video data is used in relation to disciplinary or law enforcement purposes
- How matters identified through examination of video data are communicated to patients/residents and their families
- Reconciling video data with other data sources as part of health assessments and/or adverse event investigations

Consequences and Impact

It is hugely important to consider ethical issues pertaining to the consequences and impact of new video monitoring technologies. As defined in the HFEC, this requires considering positive and negative impacts – including specific psychosocial consequences. Some consequences will be intended while others will be unintended. Further, in advance of the technology being implemented and in use, potential consequences may not always be evident. As such, where possible it is useful to document any potential unintended consequences and those consequences which require further consideration (i.e., treated as currently 'unknown'). An example of this is provided in Table 3.

Overall, the technology needs to reflect a careful balance between protecting the person (i.e., dignity, privacy, autonomy) while considering the needs patients and caregivers. Importantly, this technology will not replace/supplant the need for 'person to person' contact. Staff training will need to be a key focus of any implementation plan.

Table 3. Consequences and impact

Type	Example
Positive impacts	Promote attendance to care consistency and quality Promote patient safety Safeguard patient safety Augment carer ability Reduce staff burnout Reduce patient privacy issues/stigma Avoid abuse/harm Protect staff when accusations (unfounded) Provide picture of care event – for example patient fall, to support analysis and follow up assessment and care
Negative impacts	Changing meaning and value of work – less about human contact and provision of in person care Change in role of patient/carer/family Changing how care is delivered Changing care relationships Unnecessary monitoring of service delivery/care workers Impact in terms of privacy and changing norms for this Impact in terms of person's identity – reduction to a set of symptoms to be monitored by technology – and not a person (holistic sense)
Specific Psychosocial impacts	Reduction in time spent by carer with patient/resident Reduction in time spent by family with patient/resident Less in person time with patient Loss of individual privacy Loss of family privacy
Potential unintended consequences	Reduction in staffing Unnecessary monitoring of service delivery/care workers Potential to worsen patient/family relations (disclosing family conflicts/bad relationships) Contributing to a culture of over-intrusive assessments/monitoring impacting on patient morale and dignity
Unknowns	Impact on patient/carer relationship Impact on nature of care Contribution to a culture of self-quantification and objectification Contribution to a culture of surveillance

Ethics and Key Performance Indicators

In line with the structure of the HFEC, it is possible to decompose key performance indicators (KPI) from the ethical principles and associated system objectives. Table 4 provides a worked example of this.

Table 4. Ethics principles, objectives, stakeholders & KPI's

#	Ethics Principles	System Objectives/ Targets/Design Outcomes	Stakeholder Effected	KPI & Outcome Indicators/Metrics
1	Protect Patient/Resident Rights	Support dignity and respect Protect patient autonomy	Patient, family	Rights addressed Number of adverse events reports
2	Equal opportunities for the best outcomes for all patients/residents	Enabler of patient safety Enabler of patient experience	Patient, family	Mortiality rates Perception of care quality (staff, families, patients/residents)
3	Accountability and transparency in care.	Elicit care reporting information, so that care can be monitoring Care reporting for all patients/resident	Patient, caregiver	Availability of care reports Completeness of care reports Perception of care culture (staff, families, patients/residents) Perception of eporting culture (staff, families, patients/residents)
4	Compliance and standardization of care (i.e., reduce variation)	Enabling care reporting Enabling evaluation of care quality Enabling evaluation of patient/resident safety	Patient, caregiver	Standardization of care reports Consistency of care Perception of care consistency (staff, families, patients/residents)
5	Patient/Resident safety	Enabler of patient safety	Patient, family, caregiver	Subjective perception of safety/security Objective measure of patient safety (no of adverse events, no of potential events avoided) Timely prediction event/avoidance of event

Table 4. (Continued)

#	Ethics Principles	System Objectives/ Targets/Design Outcomes	Stakeholder Effected	KPI & Outcome Indicators/Metrics
6	Patient/Resident health & wellbeing	Enabler of active ageing/positive ageing – and allied health benefits Contributing to eudaemonia (living well) Supporting social connection and participation	Patient, family, caregiver	Health status Number of exacerbations Positive human functioning and flourishing Social capitol Personal growth
7	Positive Patient/Resident Experience	Emotional state/psychological wellbeing (avoidance of stress) Focus on ability (available capacity) Promote adaptation and bricolage Promote patient/resident autonomy Promote patient/resident empowerment Promote patient/resident involvement in care	Patient, family	Residents/patients achieve the goals they have set for themselves Subjective feeling of human agency/independence Subjective wellbeing Patient/resident feel less isolated Patient involvement in care Access to information about care Interaction between caregivers and patients/residents
8	Caregiver morale and wellbeing	Morale and wellbeing	Caregiver, care organisation	Caregiver satisfaction Caregiver burnout Staff retention Staff attrition Just culture No blame culture Interaction between caregivers and patients/residents

#	Ethics Principles	System Objectives/ Targets/Design Outcomes	Stakeholder Effected	KPI & Outcome Indicators/Metrics
9	Caregiver experience	Support teamwork and co-ordination	Caregiver, care organisation	Caregiver satisfaction Caregiver burnout Interaction between caregivers and patients/residents
10	Caregiver workload	Reduce workload Flag need for interventions where appropriate/ required	Caregiver, care organisation	Staff retention Staff attrition Caregiver burnout Efficiency Interaction between caregivers and patients/residents

Discussion

Systems Perspective and SEIPS Model

Critically, this technology needs to be specified from a human factors/system approach perspective, with due consideration to the ethical issues as outlined earlier. In line with a systems/socio-technical approach, the proposed technology must be treated as one piece of an overall solution. Other key elements include process design (i.e., how use technology as part of delivering care within framework of core clinical processes – patient/resident assessment, daily care, events reporting etc), the design of the care environment, staff training, and culture (i.e., care and safety culture).

In terms of specific technology selection and implementation, some technologies will be perceived as more or less acceptable to patients, staff and families. If acceptability issues are not elicited at an early stage in the design process, and considered as part of the design solution, serious challenges will be faced as regards implementing the system and demonstrating benefits. To this end, it is recommended that designers and developers address the different impact issues as identified in Table 4 at an early stage in the design process.

In line with the Systems Engineering Initiative for Patient Safety (SEIPS model), the proposed work system design (and allied video monitoring and other technology in use), needs to deliver practical benefits to different stakeholders. This includes residents/patients, healthcare workers & healthcare organizations. As such, it must be designed from the perspective of diverse stakeholder needs. In accordance with a HF approach, we must focus on intrinsic motivations, goals and expected benefits for these diverse stakeholder groups. These will vary according to the stakeholder groups (i.e., patient/resident, family, caregiver and healthcare organization).

Framing Benefits & Solution Implementation

When framed from a safety/risk management perspective, this technology may be viewed quite positively. The collection of data using video monitoring and/or vision systems will enable all actors to monitor and assess the biopsychosocial state of the patient and the quality of care delivery. As such, it can be used to improve operations and prevent harm (i.e., avoidance of medical error, falls prevention, self-harm etc). In preventing harm, this also protects the organization's assets (i.e., financial costs/losses, legal exposure/liability).

To deliver care in the future which adequately addresses issues of safety and quality, this technology needs to be implemented with appropriate safeguards in place. Implementation requirements will vary according to the setting and specific care culture. The primary focus should be in implementing smart solutions that leverage those who have the most impact over care quality and safety (i.e., enable caregivers). Workload and burnout are core issues impacting on the quality of care and by implication, patient experience and safety. Thus, any proposed solution must be framed in relation to addressing these issues.

Resident experience and staff professionalism are two aspects of the same problem. If resources are limited, and if caregivers are undervalued and/or experiencing exhaustion (and potentially, burn-out), then this will negatively impact care delivery. This in turn has consequences in relation to resident experience and safety. From this perspective, patient monitoring technology must be designed to reduce care staff workload and enable staff to deliver meaningful care. For example, it can augment the care-givers ability and provide protections in relation to potential care events (i.e., flag potential risks). This technology has also the potential to positively influence the behavior and actions of patients and families. With better protections and augmented care, patients and family members may feel safer – thereby contributing to relaxation and ease, which in turn has consequences both in relation to patient and care-giver behavior (i.e., cooperation and better social interaction) and patient health outcomes.

The existing AAL technologies provide many positive benefits and ethical protections (i.e., enabling independence without obtrusive monitoring). To minimize the impact on patients/residents, it is recommended that video monitoring is implemented based on the patient and/or care risk profile. Passive sensors might be in a state of 'always on'. Video monitoring/vision system might only be activated when required (i.e., in instances, where the system detects a potential event). As such, the proposed technology is 'ramped up' as needed. Moreover, video and vision systems are not stand-alone technologies. Other systems/technologies are still required to ensure a complete and holistic communications picture. As evidenced in phase 2 research, information/intelligence should be available at the point of need/care. This might include tablets for clinicians, nurses and care assistants. The provision of intelligent information to the care team as and when needed, supports care delivery. This technology might also be supplemented with bedside displays for patients. Ideally, the patient/resident and/or their family members should be able to raise the alarm if they have concerns. Further, they should have a means to report harm. Bed side tablets can also enable self-monitoring, so that the patient/resident is an active participant in their care and can focus on self-management (where appropriate).

In relation to caregiver workload and minimizing burnout, other technologies might also be of help. For example, voice interaction and/or smart language technology might be used to support care reporting.

Implementation in Different Care Environments

In relation to acute care, embedding video surveillance in hospital safety and risk management approaches, may improve patient safety, safety promotion and care culture. It is likely that there will be a stronger focus on the patient's physical health in these contexts. However, in relation to assisted living/residential settings, it is critically important that monitoring and assessment pertains to the three pillars of the person's health and wellbeing (i.e., full biopsychosocial mapping and not simply biomarkers). Long term care settings seek to replicate the environment of being in one's own home, to support social participation and meaningful connection between residents and caregivers, and to foster concepts of personal autonomy and privacy. Any technology implemented in this context should not impinge on this ethos of care and the expected 'lived experience'.

Monitoring and Quantification

The application of this system depends on an overt measurement approach. That is, capturing data and assessing the patient state using markers linked to different biopsychosocial dimensions of the person's health and wellbeing. This follows from a self-quantification approach as outlined earlier. Such an approach raises concerns relating to the objectification of the person. In this approach, the patient/resident is reduced to a set of symptoms to be measured. Evidently, the patient/resident is more than a set of markers to be tracked and evaluted. The patient/resident has an identity (i.e., a name, a story, a set of experiences, a perspective on the world, values and so forth) which needs to be factored into the design of the care process and associated technology systems. The 'face to face' interaction between the caregiver and patient/resident affords a treatment approach that addresses the person, and not simply a set of symptoms. Further, it enables the caregiver to interpret any set of symptoms. This is particularly important in relation to the interpretation of mood and emotional state, and its impact on both the social and biological pillars. As stated previously, the implementation of this technology requires careful attention in relation to the relationship between patient/residents and caregivers. In person interaction should still be the cornerstone of care and enabling positive relationships between caregivers and patients/residents.

Human Factors and Ethics Canvas

The HFEC does not offer answers for how to implement the proposed technology. It is up to designers/developers to incorporate the HFEC in their methodology so that both human factors and ethical issues are raised. The HFEC is designed to prompt discussion and critical thinking, enabling identification of potential areas of risk and evaluating the potential impact in context. In particular, the use of personae and scenario focuses attention on the people and groups affected, ways in which they might be impacted, and steps to mitigate impact. As such, it is used to build in risk assessment and countermeasures –addressing how issues are been considered in terms of product design. Arguably, in using the HFEC and raising stakeholder issues and ethical considerations, we can increase the potential for positive impact of the proposed technology and deliver technologies which properly address the 'human factor'.

Adoption of Monitoring Technologies

As the population ages, the use of self-monitoring technology (for example, Fitbits), and smart home technology is likely to increasingly become the norm. This will help pave the way for the initial adoption of patient monitoring technologies in acute and assistive living contexts. Other big drivers will be (1) hospital SMS and/or enterprise risk management systems, (2) real time hospital/event orchestration and the digital hospital, and (3) personalized medicine. As such, these trends will set the stage for the digital care facilities of the future.

The initial adoption of specific patient monitoring technologies is expected to be slow and targeted at specific contexts. For example, Emergency Room (ER), Intensive Care Units (ICU) and psychiatric settings. These settings have certain characteristics which make them potentially more amenable to patient monitoring (including the application of video monitoring and more sophisticated vision technologies). These settings are already 'high-tech' and have an existing high level of patient monitoring.

Further, in such settings, patient needs are likely to be more complex and the risk of patient self-harm and patient/staff harm is higher.

Over time, vision analytics technology is likely to become more commoditized. With an increasingly ageing population, the acuity of patient needs may increase. As care moves out of the hospital (i.e., people age in their own homes), this technology may become integral to all forms of care (for example, care in the home, assisted living and acute care).

Limitations and Areas for Further Analysis

Ideally, the HFEC is populated using evidence from stakeholder evaluation studies. In this case, no specific field research relating to video monitoring was undertaken. However, the findings of the first two studies were used to populate the HFEC and produce an initial specification for the proposed video monitoring technology. This research is being used to direct the initial prototype development. In part 2 research, this specification will be further refined. Following the analysis of field research findings (i.e., interviews, co design/evaluations and participatory sessions with stakeholders around use of video and vision systems in care settings), there will be a second iteration of the HFEC.

Evidently, there is a core requirement to further investigate issues pertaining to ethics and acceptability as part of a clinical implementation. Very often, implementation evaluations uncover important stakeholder needs and ethical issues that may not be detected without an understanding of 'use in practice'. In implementation, we will learn how best to define a solution which is responsive to diverse stakeholder needs.

Further, it should be noted that any proposed surveillance technology will be treated as a medical device under EU regulations (HPRA, 2020). Formal clinical investigations are required to demonstrate conformity of a non-CE marked medical device to the requirements of the Medical Devices Regulations (HPRA, 2020).

CONCLUSION

Older people, especially those living with cognitive impairment are a vulnerable group, and their dignity, rights and privacy must be safeguarded. Assessing the ethical implications of new technologies and/or technologies which may not yet exist and/or which may have impacts we cannot predict, is very difficult. Critically, designers should consider protections concerning potential negative consequences, unintended consequences and the 'unknown' future implications.

The implementation of video monitoring technology presents many potential positives. This includes promoting patient safety, enhancing the patient experience and reducing caregiver workload. However, safeguards are required to ensure that the implementation of this technology does not negatively impact on patient wellbeing/experience (i.e., social interaction and isolation and loss of identity). In all contexts, issues pertaining to consent, privacy, dignity and respect must be addressed. In advance of implementation, specific processes should be defined, to properly manage these issues from a socio-technical perspective. Importantly, this technology will not replace/supplant the need for 'person to person' contact. Staff training will need to be a key focus of any implementation plan.

Potentially, many of the ethical challenges specified in the HFEC regarding the adoption and deployment of video systems have solutions that can be addressed in time. Video technology has the potential to enable a safe, person focused, ethical, efficient and accountable care service, if implemented appropriately. Obtaining a holistic understanding of the ethical issues surrounding monitoring technologies will help researchers design technologies that will be effective and ethical.

REFERENCES

Adelman, E. 2002. Video surveillance in nursing homes, Alb. L.J. *Science & Technology,* 12: 821-838.

Ageing Well in the Digital World. 2020. Available at https://www.aal-europe.eu (accessed on 18 December 2018).

Anjali, J. 2008. A review of the research literature on evidence-based healthcare design. *HERD* 1(3):61–12.

Ajana, B. 2017. Digital Health and the Biopolitics of the Quantified Self. *Digital Health,* 3(1), 1.

Aspden P., Corrigan J., Wolcott J., et al., editors. 2004. *Patient safety: achieving a new standard for care.* Washington, DC: National Academies Press.

Baxter, Gordon & Sommerville, Ian. 2011. Socio-technical systems: From design methods to systems engineering, *Interacting with Computers,* Volume 23, Issue 1, January 2011, Pages 4–17, https://doi.org/10.1016/j.intcom.2010.07.003.

Beever, J., & Brightman, A. O. 2015. Reflexive Principlism as an Effective Approach for Developing Ethical Reasoning in Engineering. *Science and Engineering Ethics.* http://doi.org/10.1007/s11948-015-9633-5.

Briggs C. & Slessor, C. 2019. *Australian first CCTV trial for aged care facilities as elder abuse continues to be captured.* Available at: https://www.abc.net.au/news/2019-04-11/cctv-to-be-used-in-aged-care-homes-in-australian-first-trial/10992192.

Brown, S. 2015. *Keeping watch: Enhancing fall prevention through targeted video surveillance.* Available at: https://www.myamericannurse.com/keeping-watch-enhancing-fall-prevention-targeted-video-surveillance/

Brobst, J. 2018. *The Metal Eye: Ethical Regulation of the State's Use of Surveillance Technology and Artificial Intelligence to Observe Humans in Confinement*, 55 CAL. W. L. REV. 1.

Celeno. 2020. *Wi-fi Doppler Imaging*. Available at: https://www.celeno.com/wifi-doppler-imaging?hsCtaTracking=71993aad-fa35-441c-a26c-3a80656a9388%7Cd82d7e38-455f-4139-adec-a73be880f715.

Capurro, R. Digital Ethics. 2009. The Academy of Korean Studies (ed.): 2009 *Civilization and Peace,* Korea: Academy of Korean Studies 2010, pp. 203-214.

Cahill, J. 2019. *The Human Factors & Ethics Canvas.* Available at: https://www.tcd.ie/cihs/projects/hfaecanvas.php.

Cahill, J., McLoughlin, S. 2019. IoT/sensor-based infrastructures promoting a sense of home, independent living, comfort and wellness. *Sensors* 2019, 19(3), 485; https://doi.org/10.3390/s19030485.

Cahill, J., McLoughlin, S., & Wetherall, S. 2018. The Design of New Technology Supporting Wellbeing, Independence and Social Participation for Older Adults Domicile in Residential Homes and/or Assisted Living Communities. *Technologies* 2018, 6(1), 18 pp 1-33; doi: 10.3390/technologies6010018, http://www.mdpi.com/2227-7080/6/1/18/html.

Cahill, J., McLoughlin, S. & Wetherall, S. 2017. Lived Experience, Stakeholder Evaluation and the Participatory Design of Assisted Living Technology. Proceedings of AAATE 2017 Congress, Sheffield, UK, 12 -15 September 2017. *Studies in Health Technology and Informatics. Harnessing the Power of Technology to Improve Lives.* iOS Press. Ebook Volume 242: Pages 64 – 71. Published 2017, Editors Peter Cudd, Luc de Witte, doi 10.3233/978-1-61499-798-6-64. ISBN 978-1-61499-797-9 (print) | 978-1-61499-798-6 (online)

Carayon, P., Schoofs Hundt, A., Karsh, B. T., Gurses, A. P., Alvarado, C. J., Smith, M., & Flatley Brennan, P. 2006. Work system design for patient safety: the SEIPS model. *Quality & safety in health care,* 15 Suppl 1(Suppl 1), i50-8.

Carroll J.M. (ed). 1995. *Scenario-based design: envisioning work and technology in system development*. Wiley, New York.

Cousins, J.B., Whitmore, E., Shulha, L. 2013. Arguments for a common set of principles for collaborative inquiry in evaluation. *Am. J. Eval.* 34, 7–22.

Department of Health. 2011. *NHS Patient Experience Framework.* Available at:https://www.gov.uk/government/uploads/system/uploads/attachment_data/file/215159/dh_132788.pdf.

Desai, K. 2009. The new stars of CCTV: what is the purpose of monitoring patients in communal areas of psychiatric wards, bedrooms and seclusion rooms? *Diversity in Health and Care,* 6:45-53.

European Commission. 2020. *Data Protection: Rules for the protection of personal data inside and outside the EU* Available at https://ec.europa.eu/info/law/law-topic/data-protection_en.

European Commission. 2010. *European Charter of Rights and Responsibilities of Older People in Need of Long-Term Care and Assistance*; Publications Office of the European Union: Luxembourg.

Health Produce Regulatory Authority. 2019. *Regulatory Information.* Available at: http://www.hpra.ie/homepage/medical-devices/regulatory-information.

Holden, R.J., Carayon, P., Gurses, A.P., Hoonakker, P., Hundt, A.S., Ozok, A.A., & Rivera-Rodriguez, A.J. 2013. SEIPS 2.0: a human factors framework for studying and improving the work of healthcare professionals and patients. *Ergonomics,* 56(11), 1669–1686. doi: 10.1080/00140139.2013.838643.

Hollnagel, E. 2014. *Safety-I and safety-II: the past and future of safety management.* Ashgate, Farnham.

Hollnagel E., Wears R.L., Braithwaite, J. 2015. *From safety-I to safety-II: a white paper.*

Foucault, M. 1975. *Discipline and Punish: The Birth of the Prison.* Pantheon Books - New York.

International Standards Organisation (ISO). 2020. *Standard 6385* Available from: https://www.iso.org/standard/63785.html.

Jennings, H. 2012. Pandaemonium 1660–1886: *The Coming of the Machine as Seen by Contemporary Observers.* Icon Books. ISBN 9781848315860.

Kohl, T. 2002. Watching out for grandma: video cameras in nursing homes may help to eliminate abuse. *Fordham Urban Law Journal,* 30 (6): 2083-2106.

Miake-Lye, I.M., Hempel, S., Shanman, R. et al. What is an evidence map ? 2016. A systematic review of published evidence maps and their definitions, methods, and products. *Syst Rev* 5, 28 doi: 10.1186/s13643-016-0204-x.

Middlestadt, B., Fairweather, B., Shaw, M., & McBride, N. 2014. The ethical implications of personal health monitoring. *International Journal of Technoethics,* 5(2), 37-60, July-December 2014.

Moor, J.H. 1999. Just consequentialism and computing. *Ethics and Information Technology,* 1(1), 61–65. http://doi.org/10.1023/A: 1010078828842.

Mortenson, W.B., Sixsmith, A. and Woolrych, R. 2013. The powers of observation: theoretical perspectives on surveillance technologies and older people, *Ageing & Society* [online] 1-19.

National Centre for Biotechnical Information. 2008. *Patient Safety and Quality: An Evidence-Based Handbook for Nurses.* Retrieved from: https://www.ncbi.nlm.nih.gov/books/NBK2681/

Niemeijer, A.R., Frederiks, B.J.M., Riphagen, I.I., Legemaate, J., Eefsting, J.A., Hertogh, C.M.P.M. 2010. Ethical and practical concerns of surveillance technologies in residential care for people with dementia or intellectual disabilities: an overview of the literature, *International Psychogeriatrics,* 22 (7): 1129-1142.

Open Data Institute. 2019. *The data ethics canvas.* Available at: https://theodi.org/article/data-ethics-canvas/

Occupational Safety and Health Administration (OSHA). 2013. *Safety and Health Management Systems: A Roadmap for hospitals.* Available at: https://www.osha.gov/dsg/hospitals/documents/2.4_SHMS_roadmap_ 508.pdf.

Ouva. 2020. *Vision Intelligence for Healthcare.* Available at: https://www. ouva.co/

National Healthcare Service (NHS). 2020. *Personalised Medicine.* Available at: https://www.england.nhs.uk/healthcare-science/ personalisedmedicine/

Picker Institute. 2008. *Patient Experience Surveys:* The Rationale; Picker Institute Europe: Oxford, UK.

Pruitt, J., Grudin, J. Personas: Practice and Theory. In *Proceedings of the 2003 conference on Designing for user experiences* (DUX '03). 2003. ACM, New York, NY, USA, 1-15. DOI=http://dx.doi.org/10.1145/ 997078.997089.

Rafter, N., Hickey, A., Condell, S., Conroy, R., O'Connor, P., & Williams, V.D. 2015. Adverse events in healthcare: learning from mistakes, QJM: *An International Journal of Medicine,* Volume 108, Issue 4, April 2015, P 273–277, https://doi.org/10.1093/qjmed/hcu145.

Rickman, H.P. 1979. *Wilhelm Dilthey: Pioneer of the Human Studies,* Berkeley: University of California Press.

Rockeach, M. 1973. *The nature of human values.* Free Press. P.5.

Rozenergs, K. 2018. Available at: https://www.australianageingagenda.com.au/2018/07/04/what-facilities-need-to-know-before-installing-cctv/

State Claims Agency. 2015. *National Clinical Incidents and Claims Report: A Five Year Review.*

Social Care Institute for Excellence (SCIE). 2014. *Electronic surveillance in health and social care settings: A brief review.* Available at: https://www.cqc.org.uk/sites/default/files/CM111408_Item_8_Surveillance_literature_review_Appen_3.pdf.

Scheffler, 2. 1988. *Consequentialism and Its Critics.* Oxford: Oxford University Press. ISBN 978-0-19-875073-4.

Standford Encyclopaedia of Philosophy. 2019. Available from: https://plato.stanford.edu/entries/moral-responsibility/

The Alzheimer's Society of Ireland. 2013. *Human Rights and Older People in Ireland.* Policy Paper. Available at: https://www.alzheimer.ie/Alzheimer/media/SiteMedia/ImageSlider/Fixed/ASI-

Thomas, J. 2015. *Deontology, Consequentialism and Moral Realism.* Minerva -An Open Access Journal of Philosophy 19:1-24.

Trulysafe. 2020. *Collaborative VMS Solution.* Available at: http://vsaas.in/blog/blog_Posts/VMS_Solution.html.

United Nations. *Universal Declaration of human rights.* 1948. Available from: https://www.un.org/en/universal-declaration-human-rights/index.html.

Ulrich R., Zimring C., Xuemei Z., DuBose J., Seo H., Choi Y., Quan Xiaobo, Waterson P.E. 2009. A critical review of the systems approach within patient safety research. *Ergonomics.*; 52:1185–1195.

Webster L., Steinke C. 2009. *Evidence-based design a new direction for health care.* Design Quarterly, Winter.

Wenger, E. 1998. *Communities of Practice: Learning, Meaning, and Identity;* Cambridge University Press: Cambridge, UK.

Williams, M. 2019. *The digital hospital of the future – it doesn't start with technology.* Available at: https://www.infogoto.com/the-digital-hospital-of-the-future-it-doesnt-start-with-tech/

World Health Organization (WHO). 2013. *Health systems strengthening glossary.* Geneva: Available from: http://www.who.int/healthsystems/hss_glossary/en/index5.html.

World Health Organization (WHO). 2019. Health Systems & Services. *The Role of Acute Care.* Available at: https://www.who.int/bulletin/volumes/91/5/12-112664/en/

Wolf, J.A., Niederhauser, V., Marshburn, D., LaVela, S. 2014. Defining patient experience. *Patient Exp. J.* 1, 7–19.

Woolrych, R., Sixsmith, A., Mortenson, B., Robinovitch, S. and Feldman, F. 2013. The nature and use of surveillance technologies in residential care. *ICOST* 2013, LNCS 7910: 1-9.

Zielazinski, M. (2019). *Virtual Healthcare soon to be new presence in patients rooms.* Available at: https://www.mdtechreview.com/cxoinsight/virtual-healthcare-soon-to-be-new--presence--in-patient-rooms-nwid-51.html.

Biographical Sketches

Dr Joan Cahill, BA, MA, PhD

Affiliation: Trinity College Dublin, Ireland

Education: BA (Philosophy), MA (Philosophy), PhD (Psychology)

Business Address: Centre for Innovative Human Systems (CIHS)

School of Psychology, Room 1:18, Áras An Phiarsaigh, Trinity College Dublin, the University of Dublin, Dublin 2, Ireland

Research and Professional Experience:

Since 2005, Dr Cahill has worked as a Research Fellow and Principal Investigator at the Center for Innovation in Human Systems (CIHS), at the School of Psychology, Trinity College Dublin, Ireland. Dr Cahill has led human factors/human machine interaction (HMI) research on several European and national projects – spanning healthcare, aviation and transport. Over the last twenty-one years, Dr Cahill has undertaken research, teaching and consultancy services at the intersection of information/technologies, people and process delivery. The use of person-centered information design methodologies and practices underpins her research and teaching. Dr Cahill is passionate about human factors and specifically technology interventions that prioritise human value and wellbeing, and that positively impact society.

Professional Appointments:

June 2005 to present	Research Fellow and Principal Investigator at the Centre for Innovation in Human Systems (CIHS), at the School of Psychology, Trinity College Dublin, Ireland.
October 2010 to June 2011	Part-time Lecturer, Department of Technology & Psychology, Technology, Institute of Art Design and Technology (IADT)
October 2002 to June 2005	Lecturer, Department of Technology & Psychology, Institute of Art Design and Technology (IADT)
October 2001 to October 2007	Part-Time Lecturer, School of Computer Science & Statistics, Trinity College Dublin (TCD)

March 2002 to June 2004	Human Machine Interaction Manager, Aircraft Management Technologies (AMT), Malahide, Co. Dublin.
February 2001 to June 2001	Part time lecturer, Interactive Web Design, Dublin Business School (DBS)
June 2000 to March 2002	Senior Usability Engineer. Frontend.com, 40 Westland Row, Dublin 6.
December 1998 to June 2000	Usability Engineer/Information Architect, ebeon Ltd., Sandyford, Dublin 14
February 1998 to June 1998	Apprentice Editor, The Lilliput Press, Arbour Hill, Dublin 7

Honors:

- Winner of 'Social Impact' Award (TCD Research Innovation Awards, 2019).
- Nominated for 'One to Watch' Award (TCD Research Innovation Awards, 2019).
- Nominated for 'Social Impact' Award (TCD Research Innovation Awards, 2018).
- Over 60 first author publications.
- Keynote speaker at trade shows and industry conferences.
- Invited to share research insights in the area of Information Design, Human Machine Interaction, Human Factors and Ethics in Data Analytics, in industry led podcasts
- Travel Scholarship, 1997 (Masters Research in Philosophy at UCD).
- Research Scholarship from the Hong Kierkegaard Library, St. Olaf College, Minnesota, USA, 1997 (Master's Research in Philosophy at UCD).
- Undergraduate Exams Awards,1993 (BA in Philosophy & English Literature at UCC).

Publications from the Last 3 Years:

Publications: Book Chapters

- Cahill, J., Cromie, S., Crowley, K, Kay, A., & Gormley M. (2020). *Ethical Issues in the New Digital Era: The Case of Assisting Driving Book Chapter in 'Ethics, Laws, and Policies for Privacy, Security, and Liability'.* Intech Publishing. doi: 10.5772/intechopen.88371. https://www.intechopen.com/online-first/ethical-issues-in-the-new-digital-era-the-case-of-assisting-driving.
- Cahill J., Turney B., Wetherall S., Khan H., McGrath M., Widlicki I. (2019) Digital Transformation of Prostate Cancer Pathway and Optimizing Patient Experience, Patient Safety and Clinical Professionalism. In: Duffy V. (eds) *Digital Human Modeling and Applications in Health, Safety, Ergonomics and Risk Management.* Healthcare Applications. HCII 2019. Lecture Notes in Computer Science, vol 11582. Springer, Cham pp 3-22. https://doi.org/10.1007/978-3-030-22219-2_1 https://link.springer.com/chapter/10.1007%2F978-3-030-22219-2_1.
- Cahill, J., Tiziana C Callari, Florian Fortmann, Stefan Suck, Denis Javaux, Andreas Hasselberg, Sybert H. Stoeve & Bas A. van Doorn (2018). *Adaptive Automation and the Third Pilot:* Book Chapter in Aviation Technologies: Intech Publishing. ISBN: 978-1-78923-645-3. Print ISBN: 978-1-78923-644-6. doi: 10.5772/intechopen.70078. http://www.intechopen.com/books/aircraft-technology/adaptive-automation-and-the-third-pilot.
- Cahill, J, McLoughlin, S. & Wetherall, S (2017). Lived Experience, Stakeholder Evaluation and the Participatory Design of Assisted Living Technology. Proceedings of AAATE 2017 Congress, Sheffield, UK, 12 -15 September, 2017. *Studies in Health Technology and Informatics. Harnessing the Power of Technology to Improve Lives.* iOS Press. Ebook Volume 242: Pages 64 – 71. Published 2017, Editors Peter Cudd, Luc de Witte, doi 10.3233/978-1-61499-798-6-64. ISBN 978-1-61499-797-9 (print) | 978-1-61499-798-6 (online).

- Cahill, J., McLoughlin, S., Wetherall S., Stolberg, M., & O'Connor M. (2017). Addressing issues of need, adaptability, user acceptability and ethics in the participatory design of new technology enabling wellness, independence and dignity for seniors living in residential homes. *Proceedings of the Third International Conference on Human Aspects of IT for the Aged Population* (Part 11), ITAP 2017, held as part of HCI International 2017, Vancouver, BC, Canada, July 9-14, 2017, Springer. Berlin/Heidelberg, Germany, 2017. https://link.springer.com/book/10.1007%2F978-3-319-58536-9.

Publications: International Journals

1. Cahill, J., Cullen P & Gaynor R. Interventions to support the Management of WRS & Wellbeing Issues for Commercial Pilots. (2019) *Cognition, Technology & Work.* https://doi.org/10.1007/s10111-019-00586-z.
2. Cahill, J., McLoughlin, S. (2019). IoT/sensor-based infrastructures promoting a sense of home, independent living, comfort and wellness. *Sensors* 2019, 19(3), 485; https://doi.org/10.3390/s19030485.
3. Cahill, J, Hurley, O., and Mc Caughan, C. (2018) Addressing Teamwork Problems in Healthcare: Lessons learned from Systemic Approaches in Aviation and Teamwork Approaches in Sport. *British Journal of Healthcare Management.* Volume 24, Issue 9. pp 448–457. https://doi.org/10.12968/bjhc.2018.24.9.448. https://www.magonlinelibrary.com/doi/abs/10.12968/bjhc.2018.24.9.448
4. Cahill, J., McLoughlin, S., & Wetherall, S. (2018). The Design of New Technology Supporting Wellbeing, Independence and Social Participation for Older Adults Domicile in Residential Homes and/or Assisted Living Communities. *Technologies* 2018, 6(1), 18 pp 1-33; doi: 10.3390/technologies6010018, http://www.mdpi.com/2227-7080/6/1/18/html.

5. Cahill, J., Geary, U., Douglas, E., Wilson, S, Ferria, M, Gilbert, B. (2018). 'User Requirements & the Production of Evidence: The Analysis of Incident Data to Identify User Requirements for a New Collision Detection and Avoidance Technology to Support Safe Ramp/Taxiway Operations'. *Cognition, Technology & Work,* 20(1), 23-47. Springer, London. doi: 10.1007/s10111-017-0457-8. http://link.springer.com/article/10.1007/s10111-017-0457-8. Online ISSN 1435-5566. Print ISSN 1435-5558.

Publications: Conference Proceedings

1. Cahill, J., Cullen, P. & Gaynor, K. (2019). Estimating the Impact of Work-Related Stress on Pilot Wellbeing and Flight Safety. *Proceedings of the International symposium on Aviation Psychology,* 7-10 May 2019, Dayton, Ohio, USA.
2. Cahill, J., Power, D., Mackey, G., & McLoughlin, S. (2018). New technologies supporting patient re-enablement, wellness monitoring and staff professionalism. *Age and Ageing,* Volume 47, Issue suppl_5, 1 September 2018, Pages v13–v60, https://academic.oup.com/ageing/article/47/suppl_5/v13/5099344. https://doi.org/10.1093/ageing/afy140.66.
3. Cahill, J., Cullen, P. & Gaynor, K. (2018). 'Estimating the Impact of Work Related Stress on Pilot Wellbeing and Flight Safety'. *Proceedings of The 2nd International Symposium on Human Mental Workload: Models and Applications* (H-WORKLOAD 2018), Amsterdam (September 20-21, 2018), Netherlands Aerospace Centre (NLR), The Netherlands.
4. Cahill, J., Power, D., Mackey, G., & McLoughlin, S. (2018). New technologies supporting professionalism, patient experience and patient centred care. *Paper presented at the Annual Conference of the Irish Ergonomics Society,* May 31, 2018. http://www.irishergonomics.org/wp-content/uploads/2018/06/Irish-Ergonomics-Review-2018.pdf, pp 1-7.
5. Cahill, J, McLoughlin, S., & Blazek, D. (2017). The Design of New Technologies Addressing Independence, Social Participation &

Wellness for Older People Domicile in Residential Homes. *Proceedings of the 2017 International Conference on Computational Science and Computational Intelligence* (CSCI'17: 14-16 December 2017, Las Vegas, Nevada, USA); IEEE Computer Society. Editors: H. R. Arabnia, L. Deligiannidis, F. G. Tinetti, Q-N. Tran, M. Qu Yang. ISBN-13: 978-1-5386-2652-8; BMS Part # CFP1771X-USB; doi 10.1109/CSCI.2017.313.

6. Cahill, J., Bokser, S. & McLoughlin, S. (2017). Addressing independence and lived experience: New Technologies to Support Wellness, Independent Living, Social Participation and Community Engagement. *Paper presented at the Seventh Interdisciplinary Ageing & Society Conference,* University of California at Berkeley, Berkeley, USA, November 2017. http://cgpublisher.com/conferences/406/web/program-detail.html.
7. Cahill, J Tiziana C Callari, Florian Fortmann, Stefan Suck, Denis Javaux, Andreas Hasselberg, Sybert H. Stoeve & Bas A. van Doorn. (2017). Automation and the Third Pilot: Managing Teamwork and Workload in an Airline Cockpit. Human Mental Workload: Models and Applications: *Proceedings of the First Symposium on HWorkloads,* Dublin, June 2017. http://www.springer.com/kr/book/9783319610603. Longo, Luca, Leva, M. Chiara (Eds.) pp 161 – 174. ISBN 978-3-319-61060-3.

Publications: Conference Posters & Published Abstracts

1. Cahill, J. McLoughlin, S. (2019). The Application of Ambient Assisted Living (AAL) technologies in community living environments to promote resident wellness and safety/quality care delivery. *Talking poster at HFES Annual Meeting,* https://www.hfes-europe.org/wp-content/uploads/2014/05/Programme2019.pdf. Nantes, October 2-4, 2019.
2. Cahill, J. McLoughlin, S., O Neil, N., Nagan, N., Brady, N., Henrichs, B., O Sullivan, S., & Bokser, S. (2019). Using Ambient Assisted Living (AAL) technologies and machine learning to promote staff professionalism, resident safety and relationship

centred care in a residential care context. *Poster at 2nd Annual Conference on Professionalism,* RCSI, Dublin, July 2019.

3. Cullen, P., Cahill, J. & Gaynor, K. (2018) 'Managing Mental Health Issues in Pilots'. *Poster presented at the 6th Annual Safety Forum,* 29-30 May 2018, Eurocontrol, Brussels. https://www.skybrary.aero/index.php/Portal:Safety_Behaviours
4. Cahill, J., Power, D., Mackey, G., & McLoughlin, S. (2018). New technologies supporting patient re-enablement, relationship centred care, patient safety and wellness monitoring. *Poster presented at the Inaugural Conference on Professionalism in Healthcare in Ireland.* Royal College of Surgeons Ireland (RCSI), April, 2018.
5. Cahill, J, McLoughlin, S. & Portales, R. (2017). New technology enabling wellbeing, independence, successful ageing, and relationship centred care, for seniors domicile in residential homes. Talking Poster. *Proceedings of the Human Factors and Ergonomics Society Europe Chapter 2017 Annual Conference.* Rome, Italy, September 2017. ISSN 2333-4959 (online). http://www.hfes-europe.org/wp-content/uploads/2014/05/AbstractsRome2017.pdf.

Niall O'Neill

Education: BA English Studies, Trinity College Dublin
MSc Multimedia Systems, Trinity College Dublin

Business Address: Oneview Healthcare, Blackrock Business Park, Dublin

Research and Professional Experience:

Oneview Healthcare, various roles, 2014 – present
Deloitte, Senior Manager, 2011 – 2014
Accenture, Consultant, 2000-2006

Seán McLoughlin

Education: MSc. Strategic Management (Dublin Technological University), BSc. Information Systems Development (Dublin Technological University)

Business Address: Oneview Healthcare, Block 2, Blackrock Business Park, Blackrock, Co.Dublin

Research and Professional Experience:

Experienced product professional with Msc.(Hons) in Strategic Management and BSc. (Hons) in Information Systems Development.

I have worked in multiple industries, such as Healthcare, Insurance, Life & Pensions and Education in private and public sectors in Ireland and London, enabling organisations to develop innovative products and deliver enterprise level digital transformations.

Publications from the Last 3 Years:

Publications: Book Chapters

1. Cahill, J, McLoughlin, S. & Wetherall, S (2017). Lived Experience, Stakeholder Evaluation and the Participatory Design of Assisted Living Technology. *Proceedings of AAATE 2017 Congress,* Sheffield, UK, 12 -15 September, 2017. Studies in Health Technology and Informatics. *Harnessing the Power of Technology to Improve Lives.* iOS Press. Ebook Volume 242: Pages 64 – 71. Published 2017, Editors Peter Cudd, Luc de Witte, doi 10.3233/978-1-61499-798-6-64. ISBN 978-1-61499-797-9 (print) | 978-1-61499-798-6 (online).
2. Cahill, J., McLoughlin, S., Wetherall S., Stolberg, M., & O'Connor M. (2017). Addressing issues of need, adaptability, user acceptability and ethics in the participatory design of new technology enabling wellness, independence and dignity for seniors living in residential homes. *Proceedings of the Third International*

Conference on Human Aspects of IT for the Aged Population (Part 11), ITAP 2017, held as part of HCI International 2017, Vancouver, BC, Canada, July 9-14, 2017, Springer. Berlin/Heidelberg, Germany, 2017. https://link.springer.com/book/10.1007%2F978-3-319-58536-9.

Publications: International Journals

1. Cahill, J., McLoughlin, S., Wetherall, S (2019). IoT/sensor-based infrastructures promoting a sense of home, independent living, comfort and wellness. *Sensors* 2019, 19(3), 485; https://doi.org/10.3390/s19030485.
2. Cahill, J., McLoughlin, S., & Wetherall, S. (2018). The Design of New Technology Supporting Wellbeing, Independence and Social Participation for Older Adults Domicile in Residential Homes and/or Assisted Living Communities. *Technologies* 2018, 6(1), 18 pp 1-33; doi: 10.3390/technologies6010018, http://www.mdpi.com/2227-7080/6/1/18/html.

Publications: Conference Proceedings

1. Cahill, J., Power, D., Mackey, G., & McLoughlin, S. (2018). New technologies supporting patient re-enablement, wellness monitoring and staff professionalism. *Age and Ageing,* Volume 47, Issue suppl_5, 1 September 2018, Pages v13–v60, https://academic.oup.com/ageing/article/47/suppl_5/v13/5099344. https://doi.org/10.1093/ageing/afy140.66.
2. Cahill, J., Power, D., Mackey, G., & McLoughlin, S. (2018). New technologies supporting professionalism, patient experience and patient centred care. *Paper presented at the Annual Conference of the Irish Ergonomics Society,* May 31, 2018. http://www.irishergonomics.org/wp-content/uploads/2018/06/Irish-Ergonomics-Review-2018.pdf, pp 1-7.
3. Cahill, J, McLoughlin, S., & Blazek, D. (2017). The Design of New Technologies Addressing Independence, Social Participation &Wellness for Older People Domicile in Residential Homes.

Proceedings of the 2017 International Conference on Computational Science and Computational Intelligence (CSCI'17: 14-16 December 2017, Las Vegas, Nevada, USA); *IEEE Computer Society*. Editors: H. R. Arabnia, L. Deligiannidis, F. G. Tinetti, Q-N. Tran, M. Qu Yang. ISBN-13: 978-1-5386-2652-8; BMS Part # CFP1771X-USB; doi 10.1109/CSCI.2017.313.

4. Cahill, J., Bokser, S. & McLoughlin, S. (2017). Addressing independence and lived experience: New Technologies to Support Wellness, Independent Living, Social Participation and Community Engagement. *Paper presented at the Seventh Interdisciplinary Ageing & Society Conference,* University of California at Berkeley, Berkeley, USA, November 2017. http://cgpublisher.com/conferences/406/web/program-detail.html
5. Cahill, J, McLoughlin, S, Wetherall, S (2016). The specification of new technology to support assisted living (AL) from a biopsychosocial and stakeholder relationship perspective. Proceedings of the 2016 International Symposium on Health Informatics and Medical Systems (CSCI-ISHI), Las Vegas, December, 2016. IEEE Xplore Digital Library - Conference Proceedings Services, 2016, Notes: [*Proceedings accessed via ACM Digital Library* at: http://dl.acm.org/]

Publications: Conference Posters & Published Abstracts

1. Cahill, J. McLoughlin, S. & Wetherall, S (2019). The Application of Ambient Assisted Living (AAL) technologies in community living environments to promote resident wellness and safety/quality care delivery. *Talking poster at HFES Annual Meeting,* https://www.hfes-europe.org/wp-content/uploads/2014/05/Programme2019.pdf. Nantes, October 2-4, 2019.
2. Cahill, J. McLoughlin, S., O Neil, N., Nagan, N., Brady, N., Henrichs, B., O Sullivan, S., & Bokser, S. (2019). Using Ambient Assisted Living (AAL) technologies and machine learning to promote staff professionalism, resident safety and relationship

centred care in a residential care context. *Poster at 2nd Annual Conference on Professionalism,* RCSI, Dublin, July 2019.

3. Cahill, J., Power, D., Mackey, G., & McLoughlin, S. (2018). New technologies supporting patient re-enablement, relationship centred care, patient safety and wellness monitoring. *Poster presented at the Inaugural Conference on Professionalism in Healthcare in Ireland. Royal College of Surgeons Ireland* (RCSI), April, 2018.
4. Cahill, J, McLoughlin, S. & Portales, R. (2017). New technology enabling wellbeing, independence, successful ageing, and relationship centred care, for seniors domicile in residential homes. Talking Poster. *Proceedings of the Human Factors and Ergonomics Society Europe Chapter 2017 Annual Conference.* Rome, Italy, September 2017. ISSN 2333-4959 (online). http://www.hfes-europe.org/wp-content/uploads/2014/05/AbstractsRome2017.pdf.

Presentations: Industry Conferences and Summits

1. Cahill, J & McLoughlin, S. (2018). Quantified Wellness and Assisted Living. *Presentation to be given at the Quantified Self Meet-up, Science Gallery,* May 1, 2018. https://www.meetup.com/Quantified-Self-Dublin/events/248024937/
2. Cahill, J & McLoughlin, S. (2018). Biopsychosocial models of wellness and the human factors design of new technologies for older adults' domicile in residential homes and assisted living communities. *Presentation given at The National Medtech & Biotech Summit,* Dublin, March 14, 2018.

Sean Wetherall

Affiliation: TCG Consulting

Education: BSc Genetics/Biochemistry

Business Address: Greystones Co. Wicklow

Research and Professional Experience: Sean Wetherall is a futurist and senior technology executive with 25 years experience designing, building, and delivering cutting edge technology projects. An advocate and practitioner of Lean Startup methodologies he also consults with failing technology companies, helping revamp product lines and solve delivery problems. Working in telecommunications, mobile design and healthcare, he has built large multimillion dollar technology platforms that have delivered both functional and monetary success.

Publications from the Last 3 Years:

1. *Digital transformation of oncology pathways to optimise patient experience, patient safety and staff professionalism.*
2. *IoT/Sensor-Based Infrastructures Promoting a Sense of Home, Independent Living, Comfort and Wellness.*
3. *The Design of New Technology Supporting Wellbeing, Independence and Social Participation, for Older Adults Domiciled in Residential Homes and/or Assisted Living Communities.*
4. *Addressing Issues of Need, Adaptability, User Acceptability and Ethics in the Participatory Design of New Technology Enabling Wellness, Independence and Dignity for Seniors Living in Residential Homes.*
5. *Lived Experience, Stakeholder Evaluation and the Participatory Design of Assisted Living Technology.*
6. *The Specification of New Technology to Support Assisted Living (AL) from a Biopsychosocial, Stakeholder Relationship and Ethics Perspective.*

In: Elderly Care
Editor: Sean M. Eckstein

ISBN: 978-1-53618-446-4

Chapter 2

A REVIEW OF ASSISTIVE TECHNOLOGIES FOR ACTIVITIES OF DAILY LIVING OF ELDERLY

Nirmalya Thakur ***** ***and Chia Y. Han***

Department of Electrical Engineering and Computer Science,
College of Engineering and Applied Sciences,
University of Cincinnati, Ohio, US

ABSTRACT

One of the distinct features of this century has been the population of older adults which has been on a constant rise. Elderly people have several needs and requirements due to physical disabilities, cognitive issues, weakened memory and disorganized behavior, that they face with increasing age. The extent of these limitations also differs according to the varying diversities in elderly, which include age, gender, background, experience, skills, knowledge and so on. These varying needs and challenges with increasing age, limits abilities of older adults to perform Activities of Daily Living (ADLs) in an independent manner. To add to it,

* Corresponding Author's Email: thakurna@mail.uc.edu.

the shortage of caregivers creates a looming need for technology-based services for elderly people, to assist them in performing their daily routine tasks to sustain their independent living and active aging. To address these needs, this work consists of making three major contributions in this field. First, it provides a rather comprehensive review of assisted living technologies aimed at helping elderly people to perform ADLs. Second, the work discusses the challenges identified through this review, that currently exist in the context of implementation of assisted living services for elderly care in Smart Homes and Smart Cities. Finally, the work also outlines an approach for implementation, extension and integration of the existing works in this field for development of a much-needed framework that can provide personalized assistance and user-centered behavior interventions to elderly as per their varying and ever-changing needs.

Keywords: assistive technologies, assisted living, Activities of Daily Living, elderly population, Smart Homes, Smart Cities

INTRODUCTION

Quality of life can be enhanced by technology-based smart and intelligent assistant agents. Their effectiveness lies in their ability to address universal usability in diverse ways. Universal Usability [1] focuses on the three interrelated and interdependent areas of user diversity, technology diversity and bridging the gap between what users know and what they need to know [2]. User diversity refers to the differences in users in terms of their expertise level, age group, perceptual and cognitive differences, motor impairments, disabilities and knowledge. Technology diversity refers to a myriad of networked computer-based systems: from desktop computers, laptop computers, to portable devices, mobile phones with many screen sizes and connection speeds.

Speaking in terms of user diversity, the rapidly increasing population of elderly people has been one of the characteristic features of this modern century. At present there are around 962 million elderly people [3] across the world. This huge population of elderly people accounts for nearly 8.5 percent of the world's total population as shown in Figure 1.

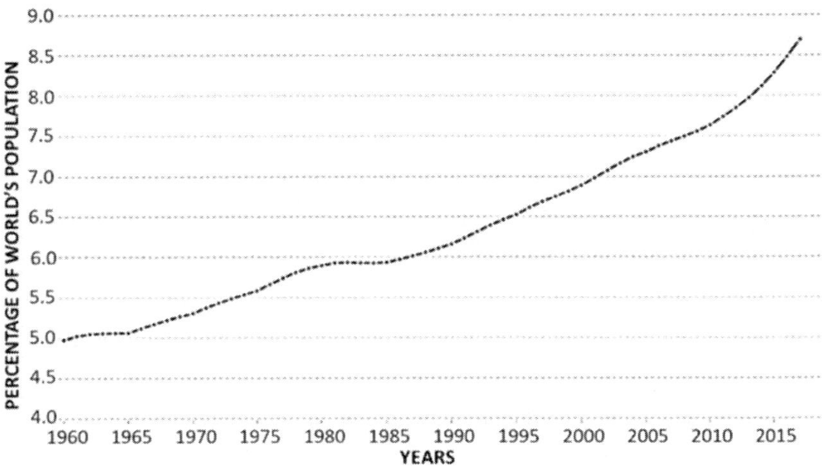

Figure 1. Elderly Population of the world expressed as a percentage of the total population.

Recent studies [4] have predicted that by the year 2050 the population of elderly people will become around 1.6 billion globally and will end up outnumbering the population of younger people worldwide. Their number is further expected to increase and reach 3.1 billion by the year 2100. With increasing age, the various needs in terms of personal, social and healthcare requirements increase.

"The United Nations Principles for Older Persons" [5] states a number of principles that may be adopted to enhance the quality of life experienced by elderly people. These principles focus on the necessity to design assistive environments that can adapt with respect to the dynamic needs of the elderly, to improve their physical as well as mental wellbeing. Increasing age is also associated with a number of health-related issues which poses an increased burden on the world economy. The number of elderly people across the world with dementia has doubled in recent times [6] and their number is predicted to again double by the year 2030, leading to approximately 76 million people with dementia worldwide.

In 2010 alone, approximately $604 billion costs were incurred to the healthcare industry in looking after people with dementia and this number is increasing at an alarming rate [6]. It is essential for modern day policy makers to develop systems and technologies that are equipped with functionalities to adapt and address these needs of elderly people. The challenges for policy makers in this context, is to design technologies that are affordable and sustainable and can help to improve the quality of life experienced by elderly people. According to recent reports of the World Health Organization, the shortage of caregivers is a major concern in this regard. The current number of caregivers across the world is only 7.2 million and their population is expected to increase to around 12.9 million by 2035, which is significantly less as compared to the large scale predicted population increase of elderly people [7] as discussed above.

Aging has also been seen to be associated with declining patterns of user acceptance towards new technologies and experiences [8]. As per [9], 40% of elderly people face some form of limitations while performing physical activities especially in the context of performing their daily routine tasks [10]. A recent study [11] has indicated a total of eight typical problems associated with aging – (1) lack of self-sufficiency, (2) prone to accidents, (3) health issues, (4) neurological disorders, (5) loneliness, (6) psychological disorders, (7) financial status, and (8) heath care costs and management. Catering to all these needs of elderly as well as sustaining their independent living [12], is a challenge, especially in face of rapidly changing households as well as evolving technology based living spaces [13] for example – Smart Homes and Smart Cities. In a broad sense, a Smart Home can be defined as a technology-based living space that provides homeowners with assistance, safety, luxury, fosters their overall well-being and contributes towards an enhanced living experience through interconnected devices and systems that operate together through sharing user data and automating actions, through an Internet-of-Things (IoT)-based environment [7].

The essence of providing technology-based solutions to address these challenges lies in the effectiveness of technology to address the diversity in elderly population which can be broadly characterized by their varying age group, gender and differences in their background [14]. This diversity in the elderly population leads to varying experiences resulting in different habits and diverse nature of user interactions. Elderly people can broadly be subdivided into two sub-groups based on their age – (1) Young elderly – aged 65 to 85 and (2) Old elderly - aged 85 and above.

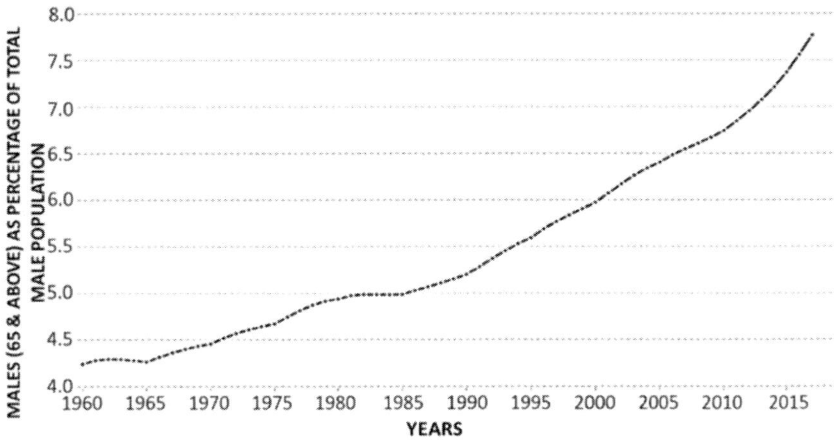

Figure 2. Males (65 and above) expressed as a percentage of the total male population.

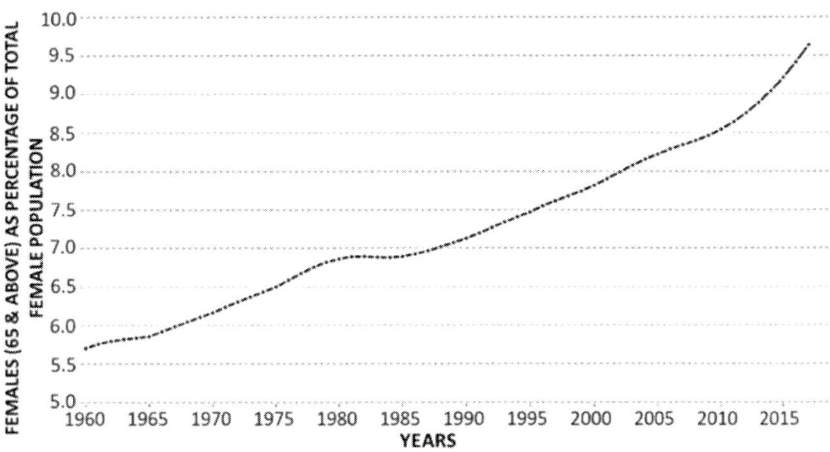

Figure 3. Females (65 and above) expressed as a percentage of the total female population.

These specific sub-groups are also diverse in terms of their gender and recent research [6, 7] has shown that this also leads to different characteristics of user interactions in elderly people. Studies on world population data [3] has shown that females aged more than 65 years account for around 10% of the worlds total female population while males aged more than 65 years account for just 8% of the world total male population. This is shown in Figure 2 and Figure 3.

Researches in this field have investigated the impact of a single or several challenges in the context of assistive technologies; however, there is a need for a study that reviews all the existing works in this field and takes a comprehensive approach towards analyzing the various challenges and limitations that assistive technologies face in the context of their implementation in living spaces for addressing the varying needs of elderly with respect to their diversities. Such a study would help policy makers and governments to work towards improving the quality of lives of elderly people and meeting their varying needs. This forms the main motivation for this work.

The concept of Assistive Technology can be broadly defined as systems and resources that take a holistic approach towards tracking, monitoring and fostering the overall health, security, safety and quality of life of its users. It can include systems, softwares, products, devices, practices as well as a combination of any two or more of these to address the needs of its users who have some form of limitations or disabilities [7]. In the context of Smart Homes, the application of assistive technologies in the future holds immense potential for fostering independent living and active aging for elderly people.

The work is organized as follows: Chapter 2 discusses about Activity Theory and Activities of Daily Living. Chapter 3 presents a review of recent advances in the field of Assistive Techbologies with a specific focus on their implementation of in the context of ADLs. This is followed by a discussion in Chapter 4 about the challenges that exist in the context of implementation of assistive technologies for healthy and independent aging in Smart Homes. The conclusion and scope for future work is presented next, which is followed by references.

Activity Theory and Activities of Daily Living

Activity Theory

In a broad manner, activity may be defined as a specific relationship between a subject (an actor) and an object (an entity existing in the world).

Activity is commonly represented as "S <-> O" which represents the relationship and interaction between a subject and an object [15]. This relationship between the subject and object is governed by two specific features – (a) subjects act on objects because they have specific needs which they seek to accomplish and (b) subjects and objects mutually determine each other in a given context.

(a) Subjects and their associated needs: Activities are considered as a way of life [15] in this objective world, which is associated with different needs at different phases. To meet these needs, a person needs to interact with objects.
(b) subjects and objects mutually determine each other: The actions of the subject on any object in a given world, depends on the attributes of the object as well as the nature by which those attributes influence the subject. For instance, if a person has to solve a mathematics problem, the person needs to have skills in mathematics. Similarly, the difficulty of the problem would determine the extent to which the person would use his or her skills to solve the given problem.

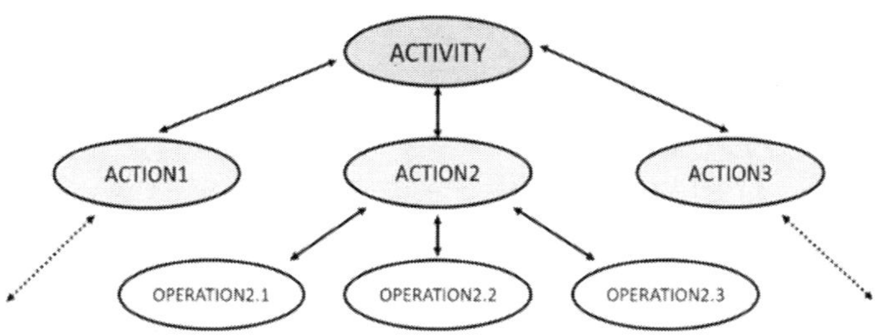

Figure 4. Activity expressed in terms of action-operation model.

In addition to these relationships between a subject and an object that determine the activity, there is also another characteristic feature which determines an activity, it is called motive. Activity theory [15] defines motive as the characteristic of an object to meet a certain need of the subject. At a closer level, it is observed that this interaction between a subject and an object does not necessarily take place in a linear manner, instead, it takes place in a hierarchical manner with needs and motives associated to objects at each level of the hierarchy. For instance, let us consider a person typing something in a specific application in a computer screen. The specific letters typed by the person are associated with the need to form meaningful words which are associated with the need to form meaningful sentences. This is further associated with the need to form collection of sentences or a paragraph and this continues. These aspects of the activity constitute different levels of the hierarchy which needs to be accomplished. Therefore, it may be concluded that needs are the governing factors behind activities.

Needs may be viewed from two different perspectives – biological or psychological. From a biological perspective, needs are associated with specific objects in the environment that causes the subject to act on them and accomplish a desired task through the activity. From the psychological perspective, needs are not associated with objects but are associated with specific states of the human body (for instance the feeling of hunger) which causes the subject to look for a specific object to act upon and satisfy this need. Activities are also not monolithic in nature. According to the initial concept of activity theory [15], an activity is a hierarchical structure which consists of three levels in the hierarchy as shown in Figure 4.

The uppermost layer is the activity that is associated with a specific motive that causes the subject to act on a specific object. The total process of the activity occurs in a step by step manner with each step leading to the motive. Therefore, it is understood that each of these steps may not directly be related to the motive but indirectly lead to it through the sequence or chain of steps. Activity theory defines these steps as actions and the respective objects at which these actions are performed are called goals. Accomplishment of goals associated with a given activity leads to the task of successfully completing the activity. In fact, actions can also be sub divided into a lower unit in the hierarchy – called operations. Operations are mostly characterized as routine processes that lead to the subject adjusting a specific action as per the given context. For instance, the action of walking might need to be adjusted differently in a side walk which is crowded, to avoid any collisions. However, recently the work based on Activity Centric Computing at Apple [16] has introduced another level called tasks in this hierarchical structure to represent an activity.

There are many important aspects in the activity theory, the following five are the ones that we consider key principles of activity theory:

(a) Object-Orientedness: This principle relates to the fact that activities are associated with objects and activities may be differentiated from each other based on different objects that are associated with them. Different needs of different subjects cause them to act on objects in their environment, specific to these needs and as per the varying motives of the subject.
(b) Hierarchical Nature: The initial concept of activity theory [15] defines activity as units of life which are represented by specific relationships between subjects and objects following a hierarchical manner of interaction as shown in Figure 4.
(c) Mediation: It is this concept of mediation in activity theory that differentiates the nature by which humans and animals perform activities. Mediation, in the context of activity theory, is mostly popular in humans. It refers to the structures and tools (for example – spoons, clothes etc.) that act as mediating objects facilitating the interaction between subjects and objects as per the needs of the subject.
(d) Internalization and Externalization: This explains that each activity is composed of both internal components as well as external components, the presence of one or both may or may not be evident based on the subject, specific needs, context and the world in which the subject is present. For instance, when children learn to count, they sometimes use their fingers for help but with time they no longer require doing the same and develop the ability to perform the counting without using fingers. Speaking of externalization, it is one of the important characteristics of human activity. For instance, a pen allows a poet to write down his or her thoughts, which leads to the activity of writing a poem.
(e) Development: Interactions of subjects on same or similar objects change with time. Activity Theory states that the nature of transformation of these interactions need to be studied to analyze

these changes to understand varying nature of activities and their associated contexts at an intricate level. Activity Theory focuses on the importance of studying these transformational patterns in activities over time for researchers however it does not explicitly mention any specific method of study as different activities in different contexts might require different methods of study.

Recent research [15] in the field of Activity Centric Computing, has added another dimension to the concept of activity which was previously broadly defined as an interaction between subject and object. This had led to the addition of another element called 'community' to the subject-object model, which resulted in a model that facilitates three-way interaction as shown in Figure 5, listed below. This work also underlines the specific nature of interactions between these components as discussed next.

(a) Structures or tools are used for the subject-object interactions
(b) Specific set of rules are used for subject-community interactions
(c) Division of labor is used for community-object interaction

There can also be community-community interactions depending on the context, specific needs, motives and nature of interactions performed. For instance, consider a user experience designer who is working in a design team to design an application for forecasting weather conditions. In addition to working on designing the application, which in this case is the subject-object nature of interaction, this employee needs to interact with other members of his or her community, which in this case refers to the design team. These interactions may be in the form of group meetings, progress updates and similar activities. Next, the design team as a community also needs to communicate with other departments of the company by conveying updates about their work and discussing further plans. This refers to the community-community interaction for this example.

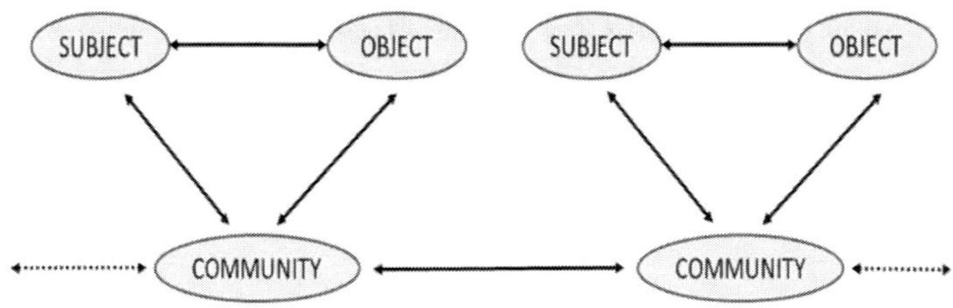

Figure 5. The subject-object-community interaction in Activity Theory.

Activities of Daily Living (ADL)

Activities of Daily Living or in short ADLs refers to the daily routine activities and self-care activities which are mostly in the context of the premises of one's home. There are multiple definitions to the exact list of activities that comprise ADLs but in a generic manner, ADLs can be classified into the following five categories: Personal Hygiene, Dressing, Eating, Maintaining Continence and Mobility.

(a) Personal Hygiene: Refers to activities like showering, grooming etc.
(b) Dressing: Refers to activities that involve changing clothes, putting on new clothes and similar tasks
(c) Eating: This refers to eating different meals during the course of the day and as per ones eating habits.
(d) Maintaining continence: This primarily comprises the activity of using a restroom
(e) Mobility: This involves the activities of moving around from one place to another as per the requirement.

The ability of an individual to carry out these activities on their own or to seek help from caregivers gives an indication of the level of independence of the person [17]. Elderly people due to their increasing age which comes with associated disabilities, are quite often unable to accomplish these tasks which increases the need and relevance to provide technology-based solutions for their aid.

Activities of Daily Living Characteristics

Based on the varying needs and motives behind a user interacting with an object or certain objects in the given context, there may be the following general ways in which activities may be broadly performed [18]:

(a) Sequential Activity: This refers to the user doing one activity at a time. When the user finishes off with the given activity at hand, the user initiates with the next activity.
(b) Concurrent Activity: This refers to the situation when the user would be doing more than one activity at a given time instance. Although these activities may or may not start or end at the same time.
(c) Interleaved Activity: Real life activities are mostly interleaved. This refers to the user starting off an activity in the middle of another activity and returning to the former after some time which may or may not be after completing the new activity that the user started.
(d) False Start: This refers to a situation like an Interleaved Activity, but the only difference is the user does not return to the initial activity to complete it. This may be because the other activity required more attention or could also be that the initial activity was no longer relevant.
(e) Social Interactions: This refers to activities that are performed by individuals in a social context. Such activities involve more than one person working towards the same goal with similar needs and motives.

Review of Assistive Technologies in ADLs

The essence of designing assisted living technologies for catering to the needs and requirements of elderly during ADLs involes accurate activity recognition. To conduct this review, we conducted an extensive search across disciplines and sources including but not limited to SCOPUS, Web of Science and Google Scholar, by using the search terms, "assistive technologies," "assisted living," "elderly people." We were able to identify more than a 100 papers that met these search categories. As the specific focus of this review is to discuss the Assistive Technologies in the context of ADLs, so we identified only those works by reviewing the literatures and the citations of each. Based on this, we were able to develop a list of 32 works which are being reviewed next.

There are broadly two major approaches for recognition of ADLs which are (i) Sensor-Based Recognition and (ii) Vision-Based Recognition [18].

Sensor Based Recognition of ADLs: With the rapid advancement of both wearable and wireless sensor systems, these technologies have provided solutions for activity recognition. These sensors collect various kinds of data and then machine learning and pattern recognition principles are generally used to infer about the activity from the obtained data. Wearable sensors provide measurements from units like accelerometers, gyroscopes, heart rates, skin temperatures, galvanic skin response and similar entities, whose data are analyzed to infer information about the activity being performed. Wireless sensors mostly provide information about the gait orientation which is then analyzed by learning models to infer about the activity which was performed by the user. However, there are two major limitations of this approach. First, real world movements are generally complex and involve social interactions, so it is quite often difficult to analyze such movement patterns. Second, wearable sensors have issues like battery life which come in the way of experiments. Moreover, the user acceptance has been a problem; people are often hesitant to use wearable sensors without having the full knowledge of the same.

Vision Based Recognition of ADLs: This approach mostly involves using cameras and computer vision principles to analyze human behavior and understand the ADLs. Different types of cameras have been used by researchers which have different functionalities that allow researches to interpret the activity. The obtained data from these types of devices is mostly in the form of frames separated from real time videos or continuous video data which contains information about body motion features, gait orientation and similar. This data is then analyzed by computer vision principles to infer details about the behavior of the user in the same.

The way these ADL recognition models work can be classified into two categories – knowledge-based models and data driven models. Knowledge based approaches mostly make use of ontologies to infer about activities. Azkune et al. [19] developed a model which comprised of multiple layers to examine human actions in the context of daily routine tasks. The structure consisted of functionalities that were related to acquisition of information gathered from sensors' that tracked user actions, understanding those semantics, and developing an understanding of activities. In Riboni et al.'s [20] work, ontologies weren't utilized to infer the particular action or task being done by the user but they were utilized to directly confirm the activity based on the small tasks and actions. They created a knowledge base of activities which included tasks and actions performed on environment variables with reasoning principles to infer activities from small actions or tasks. Nevatia et al. [21] developed a language, based on image recognition and video data analysis inferring activities in real time.

Data driven approaches for activity recognition consist mostly of various data science and machine learning methods for study of human activities. In [22], Kasteren et al. proposed use of Hidden Markov Models (HMM) to study and analyze activities. Each state of the HMM was assigned a specific task in the context of completing the overall function of recognizing user behavior and inferring the activity being performed. The model not only recognised the user actions but also tracked the rate at which these actions changed to better infer the sequence of actions related to the given activity being performed. Cheng et al. [23] proposed a multilayered learning model, based on kernel techniques to infer user actions and recognize behavior in the context of activities. They also extended this model to perform activity analysis of multiple users in the given Internt of Things (IoT)-based environment. Skocir et al. [24] developed a framework that used sensor data and Artificial Neural Networks for performing activity recognition. They tested the system on studying enter and exit events through a door in a Smart Home environment and their system achieved high levels of performance. Doryab et al. [25] used machine learning methods to design an action recommender system that would recommend actions and tasks, based on the sequence of other tasks being performed upto that point, to medical practitioners in a typical IoT-based hospital environment.

Abascal et al. [26] proposed an indoor navigation system that used multiple sensors in an IoT environment to track the users current position and help them navigate to a specific region of the environment, based on the activity they wanted to perform, through means of an intelligent wheelchair aimed to help elderly people with disabilities easily move around. They also developed a handheld device that would be useful for elderly people with cognitive impairments to better understand their surroundings and interact with the same to perform their activities of interest. An activity monitoring system was developed by Chan et al. [27], specifically for studying elderly behavior in Smart Homes. In addition to studying human behavior, the system also involved an alert system to alert caregivers during a fall. In the work [28], Yared et al. proposed a multifunctional framework which possessed functionalities to first, analyze user actions in a kitchen environnment and second, infer any abnormalities in user behavior and environment parameters to automatically detect accidents.

Kim et al. [29] developed a system to track the overall well being of elderly people in IoT-based living spaces. Their system had a database consisting of the amount of time a user usually spends in the context of interacting with various environment parameters and they developed a learning model which could detect anomalies in terms of a user spending more or less time during their user interactions with these environment parameters. The objective of this work was to study the mental well being with a specific focus on analyzing user actions and activities. In the work [30] by Deen, a host of wireless sensors and wearables were used to develop a framework that could track, record and analyze mutimodal aspects of physiological signals from elderly behavior and send alert signals during the event of anomalies in one or more readings. Civitarese et al. [31] proposed an intelligent system that could analyze multimodal aspects of user interactions to infer about elderly people successfully completing Activities of Daily Living (ADLs). The system was able to analyze user interactions in this context to understand about symptoms of Mild Cognitive Impairment (MCI) in elderly people.

Iglesias et al. [32] developed a system which could analyze the touch-based interactions of users and infer their health status. The framework also included an alert system which would alert caregivers when the users health status revealed that they needed help and attention. A similar work was done by Angelini et al. in [33], where they developed a smart bracelet to track the health status of the user which also had the alerting capabilities. As an additional feature, the bracelet could also remind users of medications and other scheduled tasks during the day, if the user forgot the same.

A socially assistive robot was developed by Khosla et al. [34] for assisting elderly people perform ADLs in Smart Home environments. They also conducted usability studies to analyze user acceptance of this robot by elderly people. An intelligent decision making framework for augmenting user performance in the context of ADLs was developed by Tarik et al. [35]. It could not only study and track user behavior but it could also recommend actions to users if they needed help completing the given activity at hand. Sarkar [36] proposed an intelligent robot called "NurseBot" that consisted of a scheduler to maintain the information about different medications that need to be taken by elderly people.

The recent works of Thakur et al. [37-50] have extensively contributed to the field of proposing various assistive technologies for elderly care in Smart Homes. In [50], the authors proposed a Complex Activity Based Emotion Recognition Algorithm (CABERA), for analyzing the emotional state of the user in the context of ADLs. Their work was able to classify the emotional state of the user into six basic emotional states – happiness, sadness, anger, frustration, disgust and anxiety. In [46-48], they proposed a framework which could analyze the user experience and affective state of the user in the context of ADLs in a Smart Home environment. In [49], they proposed an approach to analyze the user acceptance of virtual assistants in the context of interaction between elderly people and virtual assistants to help the former perform ADLs. In [42, 43] the authors proposed approaches that can analyze the multimodal aspects of human behavior in the context of ADLs to understand user performance and provide timely assistance based on need. As an extension of their works, they proposed an improved activity recognition approach in [40], that outperforms most of the other activity recognition approaches in this field and can be readily implemented in Smart Homes. In [41], they developed a system, that can track and analyze user interactions in the context of ADLs and provide task recommendations based on context attributes for helping elderly people perform ADLs in an independent manner.

CHALLENGES FOR ASSISTIVE TECHNOLOGIES

The field of assistive technologies holds immense potential for addressing the varying needs and requirements of the constantly increasing elderly population and contributing towards their independent living and healthy aging in the future of Smart Homes and Smart Cities. However, there remains several challenges, many of them are psychological and sociological factors beyond technical ones, for large scale implementation of such technologies for elderly care. Some of these as mentioned in [51] are (i) security and privacy of user data, (ii) building trust on technologies, (iii) ease of use, (iv) affordability, (v) suitable training and guidance for adoption, (vi) user acceptance, (vii) perception of no need, (viii) fear of dependence, (ix) feelings of embarrassment, (x) loss of dignity, and (xi) lack of accessibility and social inclusion.

Thus, in the context of development and implementation of assistive technologies, it is important to have a holistic view and to address these limitations for ensuring seamless adoption of such technologies for contributing towards Ambient Assisted Living of the global elderly population in the future of Smart Homes and Smart Cities.

CONCLUSION AND FUTURE WORK

This work presents a rather comprehensive review of Assistive Technologies for ADLs of elderly people. Based on the reviewed works, various categorizations of the technologies are presented and discussed. The current challenges and limitations of Assistive Technologies are also briefly outlined.

The review discusses various frameworks and systems that cater to different needs related to ADLs in discrete manners. To use Technology as a Service (TaaS) for independent and assisted living of elderly, it is essential to integrate functionalities of these systems, so that the future of IoT-based technology laden environments can address their various needs related to ADLs which include essential personal activities for Personal Hygiene, Dressing, Eating, Maintaining Continence and Mobility. Till date no such work exists that takes a holistic approach for addressing these challenges. The various challenges associated with the rapidly increasing aging population in the world, as per their diversity and their life stages, creates a looming need for development of a framework or system with multiple functionalities which could include being able to study, learn, track, analyze and respond to elderly behavior to provide personalized assistance and user-centered behavior interventions in the context of ADLs. We believe that this extensive review of assisted living technologies in the context of ADLs which includes discussion, presentation and categorization of the state of art works that currently exist in this field, as well as discussion of the challenges and shortcomings of the same, would serve as the first step for development of such a framework for Ambient Assisted Living of elderly in the future of Smart Homes and Smart Cities.

The proposed work provides a timely discussion about recent advances in this field including directions for future enabling universal access and universal usability of assistive technologies. To the best knowledge of the authors, no similar approach has been done in this field yet. This work for Ambient Assisted Living experiences for elderly people, to be provided by either human caregiver or robotic assistant or both, is to make significant contribution towards the interrelated fields of Human-Computer Interaction, Internet of Things, Human-Robot Interaction, Robotics, Data Science, Machine Learning, Artificial Intelligence, Assistive Systems, Healthcare, Health Information Technologies and their related applications. Future work would involve conducting a comprehensive review of various challenges related to implementation of assistive technologies and discussing remedies and potential measures for addressing the same .

REFERENCES

[1] Shneiderman, B. (1999), "*Universal Usability: pushing Human Computer Interaction Research to empower every citizen,*" Communications of the ACM 43(5), pp 84-91.

[2] Lazar, J. (2007), "*Universal Usability, Designing Computer Interfaces for Diverse Users*" John Willey and Sons publications 2007, ISBN: 978-0-470-027271.

[3] United Nations 2020 *Report on Ageing*, Available at: http://www.un.org/en/sections/issuesdepth/ageing/.

[4] He, W., Goodkind, D., and Kowal, P. (2016), "An Aging World: 2015," *International Population Reports*, Issued in March 2016 by United States Census Bureau.

[5] *The United Nations Principles for Older Persons*, Resolution adopted by United Nations General Assembly 1991, Available: https://www.ohchr.org/en/professionalinterest/pages/olderpersons.aspx.

[6] Bengtsson, T. and Scott, K. (2010), "The Ageing Population," 2nd Chapter in *Population Ageing - A Threat to the Welfare State*?, ISBN 978-3-642-12611-6, eISBN 978-3-64212612-3.

[7] Kon, B., Lam, A. and Chan, J. (2017), "Evolution of Smart Homes for the Elderly "*Proceedings of the 2017 International World Wide Web Conference Committee* (IW3C2), Perth, Australia.

[8] Raban, Y. and Brynin, M. (2006), Older people and new technologies, Comput. Phones Internet: Domest. *Info. Technol.* 43–50.

[9] Tornstam, L. (1996), Caring for the elderly, *Scand. J. Caring Sci.* 10 (3) 144–150.

[10] Smith, A. (2013), *Adults and Technology Use*, - http://www.pewresearch.org/.

[11] Khosravi, P. and Ghapanchi, A. (2016), Investigating the effectiveness of technologies applied to assist seniors: a systematic literature review, *Int. J. Med. Inform.* 85 (1)17–26.

[12] Barlow, J., Bayer, S. and Curry, R. (2005), Flexible homes: flexible care, inflexible organisations the role of telecare in supporting independence, *Hous. Stud.* 20 (3) 441–456.

[13] Beard, J. and Bloom, D. (2015), Towards a comprehensive public health response to population ageing, *Lancet* 385 (9968) 658–661.

[14] Seltzer, J. and Yahirun, J. J. (2014), "Diversity in Old Age: The Elderly in Changing Economic and Family Contexts," In *Diversity and Disparities: America Enters a New Century*, edited by John Logan. The Russel Sage Foundation, ISBN: 978-1-61044-846-8.

[15] Victor, K., and Nardi, B. (2012), "*Activity Theory in HCI Fundamentals and Reflections*", Morgan and Claypool Publishers, ISBN: 9781608457045, eISBN: 9781608457052.

[16] Bodker, S. (1991) *Through the interface: A human activity approach to user interface design.* Hillsdale, NJ: Lawrence Erlbaum.

[17] *Activities of Daily Living, Concept and Overview.* Available at: https://www.payingforseniorcare.com/longtermcare/activities-of-daily-living.html.

[18] Chakraborty, S. (2015), "*A study on Context Driven Human Activity Recognition Framework*" – Masters Thesis at University of Cincinnati. Available at: http://rave.ohiolink.edu/etdc/view?acc_num=ucin1439308572.

[19] Azkune, G., Almeida, A., López-de-Ipiña, D. and Chen, L. (2015). Extending knowledgedriven activity models through data-driven learning techniques. *Expert Systems with Applications.* 42. 10.1016/j.eswa.2014.11.063.

[20] Riboni, D. and Bettini, C., (2009). Context-aware activity recognition through a combination of ontological and statistical reasoning. In: *Proceedings of the international conference on Ubiquitous Intelligence and Computing*. Springer Berlin/Heidelberg, pp. 39–53.

[21] Nevatia, R., Hobbs, J. and Bolles, B., (2004). An ontology for video event representation. In: *CVPRW '04: Proceedings of the 2004*

Conference on Computer Vision and Pattern Recognition Workshop Volume 7. IEEE Computer Society, Washington, DC, USA, p. 119.

[22] van Kasteren, T., Noulas, A., Englebienne, G. and Kr¨ose, B., (2008) Accurate activity recognition in a home setting. In: *UbiComp '08: Proceedings of the 10th International Conference on Ubiquitous Computing*. ACM, Seoul, Korea, pp. 1–9.

[23] Cheng, Z., Qin, L., Huang, Q., Jiang, S., Yan, S. and Tian, Q. (2011), "Human Group Activity Analysis with Fusion of Motion and Appearance Information," *Proceedings of the 19th ACM international conference on Multimedia*, Pages 1401-1404, Scottsdale, Arizona, USA.

[24] Skocir, P., Krivic, P., Tomeljak, M., Kusek, M. and Jezic, G. (2016), "Activity detection in smart home environment," *Proceedings of the 20th International Conference on Knowledge Based and Intelligent Information and Engineering Systems.*

[25] Doryab, A. and Bardram, J. E. (2011), "Designing Activity-aware Recommender Systems for Operating Rooms," Proceedings of the 2011 *Workshop on Context-awareness in Retrieval and Recommendation.*

[26] Abascal, J., Bonail, B., Marco, A. and Sevillano, A. L. (2008), "AmbienNet: An Intelligent Environment to Support People with Disabilities and Elderly People" *Proceedings of ASSETS'08*, Halifax, Nova Scotia, Canada.

[27] Chan, M., Campo, E., Bourennane, W., Bettahar, F. and Charlon, Y. (2014), "Mobility Behavior Assessment Using a Smart-Monitoring System to Care for the Elderly in a Hospital Environment," *Proceedings of PETRA '14,* Island of Rhodes, Greece.

[28] Yared, R., Abdulrazak, B., Tessier, T. and Mabilleau, P. (2015), "Cooking risk analysis to enhance safety of elderly people in smart kitchen" *Proceedings of PETRA '15*, Corfu, Greece.

[29] Kim, S., Jeong, Y. and Park, S. (2013), "RFID-based indoor location tracking to ensure the safety of the elderly in smart home environments" *Personal and Ubiquitous Computing* 17:1699–1707.

[30] Deen, M. (2015), "Information and communications technologies for elderly ubiquitous healthcare in a smart home," *Personal Ubiquitous Computing* 19:573–599.

[31] Civitarese, G., Bettini, C. and Belfiore, S. (2016), "Let the Objects Tell What You are Doing," *Proceedings of Ubicomp/ISWC'16 Adjunct*, S, Heidelberg, Germany.

[32] Iglesias, R., Segura, N. G. and Iturburu, M. (2009), "The Elderly Interacting with a Digital Agenda through an RFID Pen and a Touch Screen," *Proceedings of MSIADU'09*, Beijing, China.

[33] Angelini, L., Nyffeler, N., Caon, M., Jean-Mairet, M., Carrino, S., Mugellini, E. and Bergeron, L. (2013), "Designing a Desirable Smart Bracelet for Older Adults," *Proceedings of UbiComp'13*, Zurich, Switzerland.

[34] Khosla, R., Chu, M., Kachouie, R., Yamada, K., Yoshihiro, F. and Yamaguchi, T. (2012), "Interactive Multimodal Social Robot for Improving Quality of Care of Elderly in Australian Nursing Homes," *Proceedings of MM'12*, Nara, Japan.

[35] Tarik, M., Bouzouane and A., Bouchard, B. (2015), "Sensors activation time predictions in smart home," *Proceedings of PETRA* '15, Corfu, Greece.

[36] Sarkar, D. P. (2018), "A Nurse Bot for Elderly People," *Proceedings of UbiComp/ISWC'18 Adjunct*, Singapore.

[37] Thakur, N. and Han, C. Y. (2020), "A Multilayered Contextually Intelligent Activity Recognition Framework for Smart Home," *Proceedings of the 3rd International Conference on Human Interaction and Emerging Technologies*, Paris, France (Accepted for publication).

[38] Thakur, N. and Han, C. Y. (2020), "An Intelligent Ubiquitous Activity Aware Framework for Smart Home," *Proceedings of the 3rd International Conference on Human Interaction and Emerging Technologies*, Paris, France (Accepted for publication).

[39] Thakur, N. and Han, C. Y. (2020), "A Framework for Developing a Smart and Adaptive Environment for Aging Population" In:

Information and Communication Technologies for Humanitarian Services, IET Publishers (To be published).

[40] Thakur, N. and Han, C. Y. (2019), "An Improved Approach for Complex Activity Recognition in Smart Homes," In: Reuse in the Big Data Era (pp 220 - 231), *Lecture Notes in Computer Science*, Vol 11602. Springer, Cham.

[41] Thakur, N. and Han, C. Y. (2019), "Framework for a Personalized Intelligent Assistant to Elderly People for Activities of Daily Living," *International Journal of Recent Trends in Human Computer Interaction* (IJHCI), Volume – 9, Issue – 1, pp. 1-22.

[42] Thakur, N. and Han, C. Y. (2019), "Framework for an Intelligent Affect Aware Smart Home Environment for Elderly People," *International Journal of Recent Trends in Human Computer Interaction* (IJHCI), Volume – 9, Issue – 1, pp. 23-43.

[43] Thakur, N. and Han, C. Y. (2018), "A Context-Driven Complex Activity Framework for Smart Home," *Proceedings of the 9th Annual Information Technology, Electronics and Mobile Communication Conference (IEMCON)*, Vancouver, Canada.

[44] Thakur, N. and Han, C. Y. (2018), "A Hierarchical Model for Analyzing User Experiences in Affect Aware Systems," *Proceedings of the 9th Annual Information Technology, Electronics and Mobile Communication Conference (IEMCON)*, Vancouver, Canada.

[45] Thakur, N. and Han, C. Y. (2018), "An Approach to Analyze the Social Acceptance of Virtual Assistants by Elderly People," *Proceedings of the 8th International Conference on the Internet of Things (IoT)*, Santa Barbara, California.

[46] Thakur, N. and Han, C. Y. (2018), "Methodology for Forecasting User Experience for Smart and Assisted Living in Affect Aware Systems" *Proceedings of the 8th International Conference on the Internet of Things (IoT)*, Santa Barbara, California.

[47] Thakur, N. and Han, C. Y. (2018), "An Emotion Recognition Algorithm for Implementation of Affect Aware Systems in a Smart Home Context," *Poster Presentation, Proceedings of the Fourth*

Annual Society of Postdoctoral Scholars (SOPS) Research Symposium, University of Kentucky.

[48] Thakur, N. and Han, C. Y. (2018), "An Activity Analysis Model for Enhancing User Experiences in Affect Aware Systems," *Proceedings of the IEEE 5G World Forum Conference (IEEE 5GWF)*, Santa Clara, California.

[49] Thakur, N. and Han, C. Y. (2018), "A Virtual Wisdom Mining 'Pan' For Connecting Retired Experts with Currently Active Professionals," *Proceedings of IT Research Symposium*, University of Cincinnati.

[50] Thakur, N. and Han, C. Y. (2018), "A Complex Activity Based Emotion Recognition Algorithm for Affect Aware Systems," *Proceedings of IEEE 8th Annual Computing and Communication Workshop and Conference* (IEEE CCWC), Las Vegas.

[51] Yusif, S., Salifu, Soar, J. and Hafeez-Baig, A. (2016). Older people, assistive technologies, and the barriers to adoption: A systematic review. *International Journal of Medical Informatics*. 94. 10.1016/j. ijmedinf.2016.07.004.

In: Elderly Care
Editor: Sean M. Eckstein

ISBN: 978-1-53618-446-4

Chapter 3

BUILDING A NEW VISION FOR NURSING HOMES IN LEBANON

Marina Gharibian Adra
American University of Beirut, Hariri School of Nursing,
Beirut, Lebanon

ABSTRACT

Contemporaneously, the ageing population in Lebanon creates a greater need for nursing services which are often provided in residential care facilities. At present, the demand for the services provided by nursing homes significantly exceeds the current supply and, as a result, the need for long-term care is increasing and long-term nursing homes are challenged to recognize and support the culture of their residents at a time when their health needs are increasing, however, quality of life remains less than optimal for many nursing home residents in Lebanon.

Despite the growing awareness of nursing home culture change in Western countries, nursing homes in Lebanon consider care as a process and have a task-oriented approach. The few studies undertaken in Lebanon on nursing home residents addressing their quality of life suggest that there is a need to place an emphasis on restructuring how nursing homes view and deliver care. Developed countries that have started putting into practice the innovative concepts of culture change, aiming at optimal elderly care, can serve as examples for developing countries like Lebanon.

However, for implementing culture change in nursing homes in Lebanon, several challenges exist; the most prominent ones being political/financial instabilities and lack of human resources: added to this is the negative attitudes of the society towards aging.

Irrespective of the existing barriers, there is an urgent need for improving the quality of life of nursing home residents in Lebanon through promoting awareness of culture change principles, and the dissemination of several models of culture change. Research in this field should be undertaken in order to provide an empirical base to guide managers and policy makers in designing appropriate policies.

It is incumbent on the Lebanese Government to find ways to invest in economic and social development targeted at providing accessible and high-quality services to its older population and ensure a respectful and independent life to the older residents.

INTRODUCTION

Lebanon, with an ageing index ranging from 41.7 per cent to 72.8 per cent by 2030, is considered a rapidly ageing country, without a national strategy or plan of action on ageing. In Lebanon, the country with the highest anticipated increase in older persons in the region, the last reported national policy was in 1994, the challenge being low financial resources, closely followed by weak ministerial coordination and lack of human resources (Economic and Social Commission for Western Asia, ESCWA, 2017).

Ageing, traditionally seen as an issue of concern for developed countries, has never been an area of priority in Lebanon. This neglect is exemplified in the health care provided for older adults (AbdulRahim, 2015). One distinctive aspect of aging in Lebanon is the lifetime experience of stress resulting from wars and political instabilities as an influence on health in late life (AbdulRahim, 2015). Moreover, among older adults, stressful reactions to the civil war were associated with depressive symptoms (Ajrouch et al. 2013).

Lebanon is characterized by having one of the highest institutionalization rates relative to the Arab region (< 5 per 1,000) and one of the highest number of nursing homes relative to the size of the older people (1.6 per 10,000 persons older than 65) (Sibai et al., 2015). At present, the demand for the services provided by nursing homes in Lebanon significantly exceeds the current supply and, as a result, the number of nursing homes in Lebanon is increasing each year due to societal demand (Naja, 2012). Currently, there are 49 nursing homes in Lebanon providing in-patient care. While essential support comes from the Ministry of Social Affairs and the Ministry of Public Health, government resources comprise less than 25% of the funding needed for such services (Naja, 2012).

Literature on these nursing home residents and the problems they face is noticeably limited since the attention to this population is only a recent phenomenon. Research work formerly concentrated on 'their problems', such as seclusion, reliance, role-loss, and poor health (Sibai et al., 2014), thus consolidating a negative description of ageing. Furthermore, sincere advocates and politicians, eager to mobilize support for frail older people projected an image of health and financial needs which emphasized aging as a period of dependency. Fortunately, such a negative stereotype is being challenged in light of the shift in the demographic trends and greater public understanding about the contribution of older people to society and their role in the family. In turn, the scientific community has responded by adopting a more positive view of ageing over the last decade. Both researchers and policy makers have shifted the focus from the negative characteristics of aging to an examination of this stage of life as a successful experience, with a view to enhancing well-being for future generation (Abdulrahim et al., 2015).

THE NURSING HOME CULTURE IN LEBANON

Despite significant national efforts to improve nursing home quality in Lebanon, quality of life remains less than optimal for many nursing home residents (Adra, 2013; Doumit et al., 2014). This is due in part to the loss of control, sense of isolation, boredom, despair, and loneliness associated with nursing home life. The absence of a sense of home, both physically and psychologically, the inflexibility associated with rigid scheduling based on staff organizational needs, processes imbedded in an institutionalized model which set disease and illness as a priority over individualized care. Despite the diligent effort of those who work within these settings, nursing homes are often perceived by media as a "last resort" (Bou Harb, 2005). Equally, the method of care employed within many nursing homes – restrictive and authoritative, is indicative of an ageist society.

There is insufficient attention to standardized guidelines and criteria for the safety and well-being of older persons in nursing homes in Lebanon, despite of the increasing numbers of nursing homes (Naja, 2012). Accreditation guidelines for the nursing homes in Lebanon are currently being developed by the ministry of Social Affairs and the standards being examined for alignment with those issued by the Ministry of public Health to ensure consistency (Sibai et al., 2017).

Whilst older people with significant support needs constitute a growing sector of Lebanese population, their voices in residential care have not been captured adequately to inform the Government's 'agenda for change' to transform services. Older nursing home residents have tended to be excluded and disempowered with neither their own voices nor those of their advocates speaking up on their behalf (Adra, 2013). The effective disenfranchisement of people in institutional settings contributes to their sense of loss of identity, lowering of self-esteem and a reduced sense of personhood (Scourfield, 2007). Older people's voices are subdued, or represented through other people's experiences and perspectives such as caregivers and professionals. Very little comes directly from older people themselves (Abyad, 2001; Doumit and Nasser, 2010).

People might argue that although residents are the best source of information about their experiences, surveying them can be challenging, given that many older residents are living with dementia. However, research has proven that even residents who are cognitively impaired can be reliable reporters if questions are carefully designed and delivered (Oruche, 2009).

Nursing homes in Lebanon provide not only medical treatment, but also a lifestyle intervention for their residents (Naja, 2012). Therefore, nursing home care should, in theory at least, be provided in a way that enhances, rather than diminishes, the quality of residential life. A real contribution to the improvement in older people's quality of life in residential settings could be achieved by culture change, for example, by helping the residents to maintain their personal autonomy by the personalization of room, having an opportunity to go out and receive friends, to cook their own meals and the maintenance of contacts with families and outside world in general (Adra et al., 2015).

Nursing homes in Lebanon can be characterized as organization-focused, having an internal quality focus; they consider care as a process and have a task-oriented approach. The resident is dependent on the care worker, there is a focus on safety and physical care, and most of the nursing homes are "hospital like" (Adra, 2013; Naja, 2012). In contrast, relationship-centered providers are described as having a focus on the quality of life of residents, families and staff, considering care as a relationship and delivering person-centered, relational care (Bowers et al., 2009; Brown Wilson, 2008; Brown Wilson & Davies, 2009; Brown Wilson et al., 2009). There is a focus on "personhood" and the relationship between the resident and the care worker, and the accommodation is "homelike" (Kehyayan et al., 2015; Royal Commission into Aged Care Quality and Safety, 2020).

The prevalent model in care in nursing homes in Lebanon emphasizes the debilitating effects of old age where staff 'do things to' residents (Adra, 2013). This devalues staff as much as residents. A more positive model is one that emphasizes personal growth for residents and staff with a shared commitment to ideas, values, goals and management practices by residents, staff and relatives (Adra et al., 2015). There is a strong focus in this way of working on the importance of relationships (Gharibian Adra et al., 2019), valuing different perspectives and fostering creativity, learning and innovation. It is based on a different level of learning within organizations, one that challenges beliefs, as opposed to imparting facts or rules.

This article provides a re-conceptualization of current practices in nursing homes in Lebanon, and an overview of culture change movement, highlighting the need for a strong vision and radical change in long-term care policy and services in Lebanon. In order to achieve this vision, it recommends a multifaceted change program. The purpose of this article is to stimulate discussion, debate, and research about a social change movement in Lebanese nursing homes reflecting the intense desire and the boundless enthusiasm of the author. The author believes that the culture change movement has matured enough in developed countries and Lebanon can learn a lot from them. While what works for one country may not be suitable for another, countries that have instituted a system aiming for optimal elderly care can serve as examples for developing countries like Lebanon. Thus, the ideas presented in this article are not intended to be a final stand on the issue but aim to instigate debate in Lebanon.

THE NURSING HOME CULTURE CHANGE INITIATIVE

In the United Kingdom and other Western countries, the promulgation of new care standards concerning quality of life and residents' rights occurred in the late 1980s (Kane, 2003). The care standards underline a number of elements including the preservation of personal dignity, offering individual choices, providing the residents with the opportunity to share in designing their care plans and to choose the way they pass their own time, participation in the management of the nursing home, and staff respect for every resident's distinctness and options (Fagan, 2003).

In response, stakeholders are attempting to shift the focus of quality improvement efforts away from those focusing solely on clinical care for single conditions to include those that focus on overall quality of life and well-being (Grabowski et al., 2014). Emphasis is being placed on restructuring how nursing homes view and deliver care embracing the central role of organizational culture in care delivery (Zimmerman et al., 2014). These and related efforts have been broadly described as nursing home culture change (Shier et al., 2014). Culture change initiative seeks to improve quality of life for nursing home residents and create a more homelike environment, by relinquishing the traditional medical model of care and emphasizing the deinstitutionalization of nursing home culture (Pioneer Network, 2017; Zimmerman & Cohen, 2010).

Efforts to change the culture of nursing homes began with the resident-centered approaches developed by trailblazers such as the Eden Alternative, an early advocate for transforming nursing homes, and the Pioneer Network, an organization that provides information and resources on resident-centered care. (Changing the culture of nursing homes, 2017). Their innovative concepts are now being put into practice by certain facilities in western/developed countries. While facilities use varying strategies to achieve change, they work toward several common goals that include:

- enabling residents to direct their care and activities;
- creating living environments that are more like homes than institutions;
- fostering close relationships between residents, family members, staff, and communities;
- empowering staff to respond to residents' needs and desires;
- promoting collaborative decision making; and
- practicing continuous quality improvement. (Changing the culture of nursing homes, 2017).

In nursing homes, culture change transforms culture from staff–centered to person-centered/resident directed, affording residents more autonomy and self-determination (Pioneer Network, 2017; Telligen, 2019), where care includes home-like choices, such as how to pass time, when and how often to bathe, and what and where to eat (Jurkowski, 2013; Rahman & Schnelle, 2008; White et al., 2012; Zimmerman et al., 2014).

Consequently, culture change is often described in the literature as a process, and as such, the term connotes a transformation of nursing homes that goes beyond superficial changes to an inevitable reexamination of attitudes and behavior, and a slow and comprehensive set of fundamental reforms (Kusmaul & Tucker, 2020; Rahman & Schnelle, 2008). Culture change proponents aim to create caring communities where both empowered frontline staff and residents can flourish, and where residents experience enhanced quality of life. Within this framework, a culture change can vary in scope and scale, taking numerous forms, including, but not limited to, cross training workers, organizing residential areas into small "households," creating environments that appear more homelike, enhancing the dining experience, soliciting resident opinions on daily routines, and writing up care plans in the voice of the resident (Jurkowski, 2013; Reinhard et al., 2006; White et al., 2012).

For example, the National Nursing Home Quality Improvement (NNHQI) Campaign (previously Advancing Excellence) promotes culture change as important to achieving eight goals that bridge medical and residential quality: restraint avoidance, pain prevention and reduction, prevention and treatment of pressure ulcers, resident/family satisfaction, advance care planning and preference-driven goals of care, minimizing staff turnover, consistent certified nursing assistant (CNA) assignment, and staff satisfaction (Advancing Excellence, nd).

Theurer et al., (2015), offer a model—Resident Engagement and Peer Support (REAP) — for designing interventions that advance residents' social identity, enhance reciprocal relationships and increase social productivity. The authors propose overturning practices that focus on entertainment and distraction by introducing a new approach that centers on resident contributions and peer support. This model has the potential to revolutionize current practice by moving from resident care to resident engagement.

A conceptual shift from resident care to resident engagement is supported by a movement towards 'culture change' that promotes quality of life in residential care and the need to rethink values, assumptions and practices currently in place (Brownie & Nancarrow, 2013; Dyer et al., 2019; Koren, 2010).

Shura et al. (2010), argue however, that most culture change comes from the 'outside-in and the top-down', rather than with collaboration from residents. In gerontology there is a growing interest in productive activity to counteract the stereotype of the frail older adult as an unproductive member of society. Here, the focus is on social productivity or contribution, as one of the aspects most threatened by aging, especially for those in a residential setting (Theurer et al., 2015).

It is increasingly recognized that staff and residents are interdependent and this needs to be considered when fostering positive cultures in nursing homes. A 'complete community' is consistent with the most positive experiences of older people and 'best care' (Brown Wilson, 2009). In a 'complete community' objectives are enablement and partnership; person-centered and relationship-centered (Brown Wilson et al., 2013); staff are working as an effective team with mutual appreciation and some blurring of roles; relatives are integral members of the team; and interdependence is an important value.

Several authors advocate that for successful cultural change the important part that each stakeholder plays must be acknowledged (Brown Wilson and Davies, 2009; Brown Wilson et al., 2009). Some commentators have suggested that models of nursing homes available today may become unacceptable to future generations (Young & Tinker, 2017). In this case, as well as for current generations of older people who would prefer something else, the shift to different options of support needs to be given more attention and determination than before, and Lebanon needs to consider the shift in all sincerity now – especially given the present numbers of older people living in nursing homes.

MODELS OF CULTURE CHANGE

Through the years, many attempts have been made to bring about a new age of quality to nursing homes. Organizations such as Eden, the Pioneer Network, and Wellspring have all provided input into creating a new future for nursing homes. Some of the better known models of culture change include the Wellspring Model, the Eden Alternative, and more recently the Green House Model (Zimmerman et al., 2014). Wellspring uses learning collaboratives in which groups of nursing homes share management expertise and approaches to training and empowering staff, and collaborative members use an outcome reporting system to submit performance data (Stone et al., 2002). The Eden Model creates a human habitat with continuing contact with plants, animals, and children and also architectural changes (Coleman et al., 2002). The Green House model most notably stresses architectural changes to promote elder-centered care in small homes; care is provided by a self-directed team that is responsible for all care and meal preparation, and collaborative decision making, resident-directed care, and close relationships between staff and residents are emphasized (Zimmerman & Cohen, 2010).

TRANSFORMING THE CULTURE OF NURSING HOMES IN LEBANON THROUGH PERSON-CENTERED CARE/RELATIONSHIP-CENTERED CARE

The western literature has addressed a variety of culture change domains that improve the quality of life of older residents (Abdi et al., 2019; Browm Wilson et al., 2013; Brownie & Nancarrow, 2013; Chisholm et al., 2018; Foundation, 2016). However, up until the reporting of this paper the contemporary research literature has lacked a Middle-Eastern perspective on the meaning and aims of culture change movement.

There is a significant gap in our knowledge about the conditions of older people living in nursing homes in Lebanon (Adra, 2013; Doumit et al., 2014; Gharibian Adra et al., 2017), and the challenge for the Lebanese society has been making evidence-based and informed decisions about everyday care practice. The policy makers, practitioners and consumer groups need to obtain a preliminary profile on the major health, social and economic problems that are encountered in such environments in order to design and shape evidence-based supportive programs that aim at enhancing and personalizing service improvement.

Existing evidence is consistent in showing that resident-centered programs require the formation of strong relationships between residents, staff members and family caregivers (Brown Wilson, 2008; Brown Wilson & Davies, 2009; Brown Wilson et al., 2009; Gharibian Adra et al., 2019), and that these relationships are built on mutual trust, understanding and the sharing of collective knowledge (Adra et al., 2015; Van Eenoo et al., 2018; Paddock et al., 2019), essentially calling for what is now called "person-centered care" (Kelly, 1989).

Person-centered approaches are founded on a rights-based approach, and embrace principles and practices of self-determination (choice and control), inclusion and empowerment (Foundation, 2014; Gillis et al., 2019; Koren, 2010; Kusmaul & Tucker, 2020; Meenan et al., 2015). The aims are to help a person get a better life on their terms and to support them to achieve their aspirations and wishes by focusing on what is important to the people in their everyday life and what support they need in order to fulfil that desire (Doyle et al., 2010; Lang et al., 2017). Most older adults take certain basic freedoms for granted, they can choose when to take a bath, what to eat for dinner, and whether to stay up late to finish a good book. Nevertheless, in many Lebanese nursing homes, residents are deprived of the right to make such decisions for themselves. Several organizations and efforts in developed countries have focused on promoting nursing home culture change where the residents' voice and choice are taken into consideration, and providing resources and networks for providers (Elliot et al., 2014; Kusmaul & Tucker, 2020; Zimmerman et al., 2014).

Few studies have been undertaken in Lebanon exploring the meaning of quality of life from, the standpoint of the older residents, and from other key stakeholders. In 2015, Adra et al. constructed a quality of life model that integrated the views of older residents, staff members and family caregivers. The emergent model indicated that a culture strongly based on residents' choice leads to positive resident outcomes. For instance, being able to say what the resident means without fear has been linked to maintaining the personhood and the identity of the older resident. The important features highlighted in the model were to have, choice, control and voice; and increased participation in decision making by the nurses and family caregivers were linked to lowering prevalence of feelings of loneliness among residents. On the other hand, failure of staff members to involve residents in realizing their choices, in addition to conflicts between what the residents want and what the managers believe they need, were identified as factors hindering the quality of life of the older residents (Adra et al., 2015). Moreover, staff members believed that residents have the right to be actively involved in the planning of their care, to make informed decisions and exercise choice and control over the services they receive. Conversely, specifying work procedures and rules in combination with surveillance was linked to higher prevalence of complications and immobility. Older residents expressed their preference for the environment to be home-like, enhancing their dignity and respect, their needs and desires to be met in terms of waking up and going to sleep, dining, dressing, bathing, etc. (Adra et al., 2015, Gharibian Adra et al., 2017).

In order to identify the concerns of the older resident, thereby, facilitating the delivery of person-centered, compassionate care, ensuring positive relationships in nursing home in Lebanon was found to be crucially important (Gharibian Adra, 2019). One of the quality of life domains identified by Van Leeuwen et al., (2019), Adra et al., (2015), Brown Wilson, (2009) was having close relationships with staff, which makes them feel supported and enable them to mean something for others. Ensuring a good quality of life in these institutions and promoting positive relationships with the staff in nursing homes can mitigate the adverse effects of institutionalization in older adults.

Doyle et al., (2010) identified the "What matters to you" (WMTY) approach that promotes compassionate relationship-centered care (Dewar & Nolan 2013) and supports this concept. It involves introducing a change in practice, whereby, nursing staff ask about what is important to the resident, rather than simply concentrating on their diagnosis and medical history. The approach suggests that to provide compassionate care we need to know the details of care that matter to the older person (Health Foundation 2014). Information captured through this approach provides staff with a unique knowledge of the life of the person (Lown et al., 2011), which then informs the plan of care for that resident. Moreover, compassionate care involves developing a relationship of equals where the caregiver conveys an understanding of the resident's concerns in a way that alleviates some of those concerns (Burnell & Agan, 2013; Von Dietze & Orb 2000). There is a critical link between services who regard the resident as an equal contributor to their care, where their opinions are sought and valued, and the provision of compassionate relationship-centered care (England, 2014; Gharibian Adra et al., 2019; Tierney et al., 2019).

Therefore, if care will truly be provided with compassion and dignity, sustaining interpersonal relationships is essential. In order to achieve these goals administrators and managers of nursing homes should facilitate ongoing conversations between stakeholders, and that nursing staff include all perspectives in these conversations (Kusmaul & Tucker, 2020). In order to make culture change a reality, "staff reinforcement, staff deliberation, stakeholder collaboration, and supportive leadership" (Palmer et al., 2018, p. 275) are essential. Direct care workers need ongoing mentoring to negotiate nuances between choice and care, such as the regular culture change meetings and an environment where they feel safe enough to address their challenges.

The few studies undertaken in Lebanon on nursing home residents addressing their quality of life suggest that there is a need to place an emphasis on restructuring how nursing homes view and deliver care. Developed countries that have started putting into practice the innovative concepts of culture change, aiming at optimal elderly care, can serve as examples for developing countries like Lebanon. There is an urgent need for improving the quality of life of nursing home residents in Lebanon through promoting awareness of culture change principles, and the dissemination of several models of culture change. Commissioning very traditional models of care that reflect deeply embedded assumptions and beliefs about what's 'appropriate', practical and affordable need to be halted, and these assumptions need to be openly discussed in order to widen choice, increase control and strengthen voice.

Challenges/Barriers to Achieving the Vision in Nursing Homes

Recent evaluations point to challenges in implementing person-centered/relationship centered philosophies (Edvardson et al., 2010; Edvardson et al., 2008).

1) Lack of clear steps to initiate change, the lack of consistent terminology, philosophical differences surrounding the practical and tangible changes necessary to change culture.

2) Culture change movement is being built largely around innovations, the changes are mostly not evidence-based, and their outcomes somewhat uncertain. Published studies do not provide sufficient evidence to guide nursing homes or governing bodies to make informed decisions in the implementation of culture change to best improve the quality of life in nursing homes (Zimmerman et al., 2014).
3) Ageism and other forms of discrimination.
4) A failure of staff members to involve residents in realizing their choices, conflicts between what the residents want and what the case managers believe they need.
5) One of the challenges of transforming the nursing home culture is how much choice is realistic in a setting where the needs of multiple frail older residents, and residents living with dementia have to be met. When medical and safety needs conflict with preferences, facilities should consider using a person-centered planning approach (Behrens et al., 2018) to negotiate choices that are perceived unsafe.
6) Difficulty in supplying and maintaining adequate staffing, materials and equipment.

The unique historical, political, security, and economic issues of Lebanon influence the experience of nursing home residents. At present Lebanon is encountering additional challenges that make the implementation of culture change difficult. Added to this is the limited resources to transform and sustain a culture of community over time.

The challenges facing Lebanon can be grouped into Political/financial instabilities and lack of human resources.

1) Political and financial instabilities and unique economic circumstances in Lebanon affect the well-being of the Lebanese vulnerable older population. The absence of health coverage for older people remains the main concern and most pressing barrier to the well-being of older persons.

2) Lack of political will and legislation, lack of financial resources, the absence of guidelines for old-age homes and the rising cost of medical and health-care services, the need for additional resources rather than possibilities and hopes for a different future that need resourcing.
3) In Lebanon, conversations about a vision for a good life in nursing homes can be difficult because there is currently no visible discussion going on around rights, equality and opportunities for this population of older people.
4) The invisibility, isolation and 'societal neglect' of older people with high support needs, very low awareness of and understanding about – and possibly lack of support for an independent living ethos for this population of older people;
5) Caring for older adults is given a low status and may hold negative social and ageist attitudes.
6) Limited number of professional nurses specialized in gerontological nursing, having the ability to deliver individualized, high-quality care. The current focus remaining on the provision of care mainly by nursing assistants.
7) Limited number of leaders having the ability to create change from institutional to individualized care on a large scale, and having the ability to offer such education and training to support change.

Recommendations for a Vision for a Good Life in Nursing Homes in Lebanon

While there are many shortcomings to the care of nursing home residents in Lebanon, the author remains a strong believer that the care of an older resident goes far beyond financial support and official government input.

1) There is an urgent need to improve Lebanese national standards and regulations applicable to nursing home residents to allow for the fulfillment of resident's care needs by professional nurses and other personnel specialized in elderly care.
2) We need to change the way we think about older people; a paradigm shift in our conceptual approach to aging is needed recognizing the importance of person-centered approach to aging and the role of determinants of quality of life in nursing homes.
3) Develop awareness campaigns that challenge and overcome the current stigma about ageism.
4) There is an urgent need to increase the number of nursing staff with higher educational background and other specialists in the area of elderly care. The availability of trained and well-motivated staff to meet the needs of residents in nursing homes is essential to implement culture change.
5) Provide postgraduate training and continuing education in these fields. Such steps will promote health education on older people, which in turn improves the quality of health care and quality of life of the residents.
6) There is a need for strengthening institutional arrangements on aging and for promoting knowledge production, which meets policy-relevant priorities.
7) Bringing the academic community together with policy makers, practitioners and service users to facilitate discussion about research and developments within the nursing home industry to shape the future in this area of health and social care provision. This relationship needs to be strengthened and developed in mutual collaboration in order to put forward a set of approaches for sharing, exploring and embedding this vision. This includes nursing leaders, who favor promoting a compassionate culture, in which staff feel psychologically safe, are able to take appropriate risks, and are open to change (West et al., 2017).
8) Willingness of researchers, practitioners, policy makers, and service users to ensure the vision becomes a reality, with the older people's

voices raised, heard and responded to at every level. It has been noted that compassion/person centered care requires a facilitative environment to flourish (Tierney et al., 2019). When unable to deliver care in a way they would wish, due to external pressures, health professionals can encounter 'moral distress' (Mauno, et al., 2016), undertaking their work in an efficient manner but not connecting with patients.

9) The creation of multidisciplinary networks at the national, regional, and international levels enhancing the quality of research and care related to the ageing population. This change would involve a significant move towards thinking explicitly about what older people who need a lot of support in their lives would like their lives to be like and about the support that would help them to experience this. By critically reviewing current practice and opening up to creative ideas, a broader range of support could be planned, designed, and provided.

10) Nursing homes that import culture change are likely to achieve better results if they stay alert to potential implementation pitfalls, which they can then work to resolve. This understanding thus empowers providers, making success more likely. A listening, proactive style of management is more likely to encourage open relationships and empower staff to be creative.

RECOMMENDATIONS FOR RESEARCH

Nursing home culture change remains an evolving field. Although culture change has clear face validity, the current evidence does not give providers sufficient information for selecting interventions based on the expectation of improving outcomes. Rigorous research on implementation and outcomes of culture change is needed to determine the specific impact of culture change on quality of life and to provide guidance to providers and policy makers (Grabowski et al., 2014); research should examine whether and which models/components of culture change relate to clinically significant quality of life outcomes (Rahman & Schnelle 2008). Such findings would provide the credibility needed to advance the culture change movement to the next level (Shier et al., 2014).

Among the first interventions to consider for study can be those that increase resident choice over daily activities since resident choice is a core value within the culture change movement (Shier et al., 2014). Future studies should carefully measure the process of implementation and fidelity to the culture change intervention to improve understanding of the extent to which changes in intervention outcomes can be attributed to change in nursing home culture.

CONCLUSION

Despite the political and financial instabilities, quality of life in nursing homes in Lebanon is gaining prominence in due to heightened awareness of the issue. The Centre for Studies on Ageing in Lebanon has set the prime objectives of shedding more light on older adult issues at the domestic and regional levels and persuading policy makers and funders to prioritize ageing. As stated earlier, Lebanese nursing homes place greater emphasis on tasks rather than on the residents as persons. It is hoped that the findings of the scarce number of studies undertaken in Lebanon addressing the quality of life of nursing home residents (Adra et al., 2015; Gharibian Adra et al., 2017; Gharibian Adra et al., 2018; Gharibian Adra et al., 2019) will draw the attention of administrators, nursing staff, and policy-makers and will bring about cultural transformations leading to the perception of older residents as individuals and to improve flexibility in care delivery. Service needs to be increasingly centered on the residents based on consultation, independence, making selections, personal care, and resident participation in decision-making (Adra et al., 2015, Gharibian Adra et al., 2017). The shift in nursing home culture toward the resident-centered approach to care could establish a future trend. This implies that policy makers, nursing management, and staff members should embrace change and define their roles in the context of advancing the quality of life of the older residents.

Nursing homes should not be seen as places where older individuals die, but as places where they live and lead a decent life (Murphy et al., 2006).

The author is fully aware of the challenges facing the operationalization of the concepts presented in this article, as Lebanon remains vulnerable to internal political instabilities which threaten the ability to address the needs of its older population in general and the needs of nursing home residents in particular. It is incumbent on the Lebanese Government to find ways to invest in economic and social development targeted at providing accessible and high-quality services to its older population and ensure a respectful and independent life to the older residents. "Senior citizens are not a problem but a joy, and improving their quality of life is a genuinely noble purpose" (Milliband, 2001 p. 18).

References

Abdi, S., Spann, A., Borilovic, J., de Witte, L., & Hawley, M. (2019). Understanding the care and support needs of older people: a scoping review and categorization using the WHO international classification of functioning, disability and health framework (ICF). *BMC geriatrics,* 19(1), 195.

Abdulrahim, S., Ajrouch, K. J., Jammal, A., & Antonucci, T. C. (2015). Aging in Lebanon: Challenges and Opportunities. *The Gerontologist,* 55 (4), 511-518.

Abyad, A. (2001). Health care for older persons: A country profile – Lebanon. *Journal of the American Geriatrics Society,* 49, 1366-1370.

Adra, M. (2013). *Generating a model of quality of life for older nursing home residents in the Lebanon: A grounded theory study*. University of Manchester.

Adra, M. G., Hopton, J., & Keady, J. (2015). Constructing the meaning of quality of life for residents in care homes in the Lebanon: perspectives of residents, staff and family. *International Journal of Older People Nursing,* 10(4), 306-318.

Advancing Excellence in America's Nursing Homes. (nd). *Eight goals.* Retrieved July 1, 2020, from: https://www.healthleadersmedia.com/clinical-care/advancing-excellence-americas-nursing-homes.

Ajrouch, K. J., Abdulrahim, S., & Antonucci, T. C. (2013) Stress, social relations, and psychological well-being over the life course: a focus on Lebanon, *GeroPsych. The Journal of Gerontopsychology and Geriatric Psychiatry*, 26, 15–28. doi: 10.1024/1662–9647/a000076.

Behrens, L., Van Haitsma, K., Brush, J., Boltz, M., Volpe, D., & Kolanowski, A. M. (2018). Negotiating risky preferences in nursing homes: A case study of the Rothschild person-centered care planning approach. *Journal of gerontological nursing,* 44(8), 11-17.

Bou Harb, R. (2005). Chronique Sociales. *Annales, Travail Social et Recherche*, *7*(21), 2004-2005. Beirut: Universite Saint-Joseph.

Bowers, H., Clark, A., Crosby, G., Easterbrook, L., Macadam, A., MacDonald, R., Macfarlane, A., Maclean, M., Patel, M., Runnicles, D., Oshinaike, T. and Smith, C. (2009). *A research project exploring the voice, choice and control of older people with high support needs.* Commissioned by the Joseph Rowntree Foundation's Independent Living Committee.

Brown Wilson, C., Swarbrick, C., Pilling, M., & Keady, J. (2013). The senses in practice: enhancing the quality of care for residents with dementia in care homes. *J Adv Nurs,* 69(1), 77-90.

Brown Wilson, C. (2008). Using relationships to develop practice that values the contribution of older people, families and staff. International *Journal of Older People Nursing,* 3(4), 274-277.

Brown Wilson, C. & Davies, S. (2009). Developing relationships in long term care environments: the contribution of staff. *Journal of clinical nursing,* 18(12), 1746-1755. 4.

Brown Wilson, C. Davies, S., & Nolan, M. (2009). Developing personal relationships in care homes: realizing the contributions of staff, residents and family members. *Ageing and Society,* 29(7), 1041-1063.

Brown Wilson, C. (2009). Developing community in care homes through a relationship-centered approach. *Health and Social Care in the Community,* 17 (2), 177-186.

Brownie, S., & Nancarrow, S. (2013). Effects of person-centered care on residents and staff in aged-care facilities: a systematic review. *Clinical interventions in Aging,* 8, 1.

Burnell, L., & Agan, D. L. (2013). Compassionate care: Can it be defined and measured? The development of the Compassionate Care Assessment Tool. *International Journal of Caring Sciences,* 6(2), 180-187.

Changing the Culture of Nursing Homes, M. H. 2017. (n.d.). *The commonwealth fund.* Issue of the Month.

Chisholm, L., Zhang, N. J., Hyer, K., Pradhan, R., Unruh, L., & Lin, F. C. (2018). Culture change in nursing homes: What is the role of nursing home resources? *INQUIRY: The Journal of Health Care Organization, Provision, and Financing,* 55, 0046958018787043.

Dewar, B., & Nolan, M. (2013). Caring about caring: Developing a model to implement compassionate relationship centred care in an older people care setting. *International journal of nursing studies,* 50(9), 1247-1258.

Doumit, J. H., Nasser, R. N., & Hanna, D. R. (2014). Nutritional and health status among nursing home residents in Lebanon: comparison across gender in a national cross sectional study. *BMC Public Health,* 14(1), 629.

Doumit, J., & Nasser, R. (2010). Quality of life and wellbeing of the elderly in Lebanese nursing homes. *International Journal of Health Care Quality Assurance,* 23(1), 72-93.

Doyle, C., Reed, J., Woodcock, T., & Bell, D. (2010). Understanding what matters to patients–identifying key patients' perceptions of quality. *JRSM short reports,* 1(1), 1-6.

Dyer SM, Valeri M, Arora N, Ross T, Winsall M, Tilden D, Crotty M. (2019). *Review of International Systems for Long-Term Care of Older People.* Flinders University, Adelaide, Australia.

Economic and Social Commission for Western Asia. (2017). *Ageing in ESCWA Member States Third Review and Appraisal of the Madrid International Plan of Action on Ageing* (12). United Nations Beirut. https://www.unescwa.org/publications/ageing-escwa-member-states.

Eden Alternative: Findings after 1 year of implementation. *Journal of Gerontology: Medical Sciences*, *57*, M422–M427. Retrieved from http://dx.doi.org/10.1093/gerona/57.7.M422.

Edvardsson D., Winblad B. & Sandman P. O. (2008) Person centered care for people with severe Alzheimer's disease – current status and ways forward. *The Lancet Neurology* 7, 362–367.

Edvardsson, D., Fetherstonhaugh, D., Nay, R. (2010). Promoting a continuation of self and normality: person-centered care as described by people with dementia, their family members and aged care staff. *Journal of Clinical Nursing*. 19 (17-18), 2611-2618. https://doi.org/10.1111/j.1365-2702.2009.03143.x.

Elliot, A.Cohen, L. W., Reed, D., Nolet, K., Zimmerman, S. (2014). A "recipe" for culture change? Findings from the THRIVE survey of culture change adopters. *The Gerontologist,* 54(Suppl. 1), S17–S24. doi: 10.1093/geront/gnt133.

England, N. (2014). *Safe, compassionate care for frail older people using an integrated care pathway*. Redditch: NHS England.

Fagan, R. M. (2003). Pioneer Network: Changing the culture of aging in America. *Journal of Social Work in Long-Term Care,* 2,125–140. Retrieved from http://dx.doi.org/10.1300/J181v02n01_09.

Foundation, H. (2014). *Person-centred care made simple: what everyone should know about person-centred care*: *Health Foundation*.

Foundation, H. (2016). *Staffing matters; funding counts—Pressure point: Associate nurses*.

Gharibian Adra, M., Aharonian, Z., & Sibai, A. M. (2019). Exploring resident-staff relationships in nursing homes in Lebanon. *International journal of qualitative studies on health and well-being,* 14(1), 1688605.

Gharibian Adra, M., Hopton, J., Keady, J. (2017) "Nursing home quality of life in the Lebanon," *Quality in Ageing and Older Adults,* 18 (2), pp.145-156, https://doi.org/10.1108/QAOA-01-2016-0002.

Gharibian, Adra, M., Hopton, J., Keady, J. (2018). Generating a Model of Quality of Life for Older Nursing Home Residents in Lebanon: A Grounded Theory Study. In D. L. Nielsen (Ed.), *Elderly Care, Options, Challenges and Trends.* (pp.1-26). Nova Science Publishers: New York.

Gillis, K., Lahaye, H., Dom, S., Lips, D., Arnouts, H., & Van Bogaert, P. (2019). A person-centred team approach targeting agitated and aggressive behavior amongst nursing home residents with dementia using the Senses Framework. *International Journal of Older People Nursing,* 14(4), e12269.

Grabowski, D. C., O'Malley, A. J., Afendulis, C. C., Caudry, D. J., Elliot, A., & Zimmerman, S. (2014). Culture change and nursing home quality of care. *The Gerontologist,* 54(Suppl_1), S35-S45.

Jurkowski, E. T. (2013). *Implementing culture change in long-term care: Benchmarks and strategies for management and practice*: Springer Publishing Company.

Kane, R. A., Kling, K. C., Bershadsky, B., Kane, R. L., Giles, K., Degenholtz, H. B., Cutler, L. J. (2003). Quality of life measures for nursing home residents. *The Journals of Gerontology Series A: Biological Sciences and Medical Sciences,* 58(3), M240-M248.

Keane, B. (2004). Building the new culture of aging--One leader at a time. *Nursing Homes Long Term Care Management,* 53(8), 44-46.

Kehyayan, V., Hirdes, J. P., Tyas, S. L., & Stolee, P. (2015). Residents' self-reported quality of life in long-term care facilities in Canada. *Canadian Journal on Aging,* 34(2), 149–164.

Kelly, M. (1989).The Omnibus Budget Reconciliation Act of 1987. A policy analysis. *Nursing Clinics of North America,* 24, 791794.

Koren, M. J. (2010). Person-centered care for nursing home residents: The culture-change movement. *Health Affairs,* 29(2), 312-317.

Kunkel, S. R. (2006). *Consumer voice and choice in long-term care*: Springer Publishing Company.

Kusmaul, N., & Tucker, G. G. (2020). Person-Centered Care in Nursing Homes: Many Stakeholders, Many Perspectives. *Journal of Gerontological Nursing,* 46 (5), 9-13.

Lang, D., Hoey, C., Whelan, M., & Price, G. (2017). The introduction of "What Matters to You": a quality improvement initiative to enhance compassionate person-centered care in hospitals in Ireland. *Int J Integr Care,* 17(5), 445.

Lown, B. A., Rosen, J., & Marttila, J. (2011). An agenda for improving compassionate care: a survey shows about half of patients say such care is missing. *Health Affairs,* 30(9), 1772-1778.

Lung, C. C., & Liu, J. Y. W. (2016). How the perspectives of nursing assistants and frail elderly residents on their daily interaction in nursing homes affect their interaction: a qualitative study. *BMC geriatrics,* 16(1), 13.

Mauno, S., Ruokolainen, M., Kinnunen, U., Bloom, J. (2016). Emotional labor and work engagement among Finnish nurses: Examining perceived compassion, leadership and work ethic as stress buffers. *Journal of Advanced Nursing.* 72. 10.1111/jan.12906.

Meenan, H., Rees, N., & Doron, I. (2015). *Towards human rights in residential care for older persons: international perspectives*: Routledge.

Miliband, D. (2001). Growing older: Research and policy. *The Growing Older Programme Occasional.* Paper 1 presented at the Launch Conference (pp.18).

Murphy, K., O'Shea, E., Cooney, A., Shiel, A., & Hodgins, M. (2006). *Improving quality of life for older people in long-stay care settings in Ireland* (Rep. No. 93). Dublin: National Council on Ageing and Older People.

Naja, N. (2012). Long term stay institutions in Lebanon. *Lebanese Medical Journal,* 103(369), 1-5.

Network, P. (2017). *What is culture change*. nd. In.

Oruche, M. U. (2009). Research With Cognitively Impaired Participants. *J Nurs Law;* 13(3).

Paddock, K., Brown Wilson, C., Walshe, C., & Todd, C. (2019). Care home life and identity: A qualitative case study. *The Gerontologist,* 59(4), 655-664.

Palmer, J. A., Parker, V. A., Berlowitz, D., Snow, A. L., & Hartmann, C. W. (2018). Resident choice: a nursing home staff perspective on tensions and resolutions. *Geriatric Nursing,* 39(3), 271-278.

Rahman, A. N., & Schnelle, J. F. (2008). The nursing home culture-change movement: Recent past, present, and future directions for research. *The Gerontologist,* 48(2), 142-148.

Reinhard, S. C., Howell White, S., Quinn, W. (2006). Choice and Institutionalized Elderly. In S. Kunkel & V. Wellin (Eds.), *Consumer Voice and Choice in Long-Term Care.* (pp. 21-42). Springer publishing: New York.

Royal Commission into Aged Care Quality and Safety. (2020). *Review of International Systems for Long-Term Care of Older People.* Research paper 2. Commonwealth of Australia. https://agedcare.royal commission.gov.au/publications/Documents/research-paper-2-review-international-systems-long-term-care.pdf.

Scourfield, P. (2007). Helping older people in residential care remain full citizens. *British Journal of Social Work,* 37(7), 1135-1152.

Shier, V., Khodyakov, D., Cohen, W. L., Zimmerman, S., and Saliba, D (2014). What Does the Evidence Really Say About Culture Change in Nursing Homes? *The Gerontologist,* 54, S1-S7.

Shura, R., Rebecca, S., and Dale, D. (2010). Culture Change in Long-Term Care: Participatory Action Research and the Role of the Resident. *The Gerontologist.* 51. 212-25. 10.1093/geront/gnq099.

Sibai, A., Rizk, A., & Kronfol, N. (2014). *Ageing in the Arab region: Trends, implications and policy options.* Center for Studies on Aging (CSA), ESCWA and UNFPA. Retrieved from http://csa.org. lb/cms/assets/csa% 20publications/unfpa, 20.

Sibai, A. M., Rizk, A., Costanian, C., & Beard, J. R. (2017). Landscape of research on older adults' health in the Arab region: Is it demography-driven or development-dependent? *Journals of Gerontology Series B: Psychological Sciences and Social Sciences,* 72(4), 680-687.

Sibai, A. M., Rizk, A., & Kronfol, N. M. (2015). Aging in Lebanon: perils and prospects. *Lebanese Medical Journal,* 103(1716), 1-6.

Stone, R. I., Reinhard, S. C., Bowers, B. Zimmerman, D., Phillips, C. D. Hawes, C., . . . Jacobson, N. (2002). Evaluation of the Wellspring model for improving nursing home quality. *The Commonwealth Fund.* Retrieved from http://www.commonwealthfund.org/~/media/Files/

Publications/Fund%20Report/2002/Aug/Evaluation%20of%20the%20 Wellspring%20Model%20for%20Improving%20Nursing%20Home% 20Quality/stone_wellspringevaluation%20pdf.pdf.

Telligen. (2019). *Change Packages to Support the National Nursing Home Quality Care Collaborative (NNHQCC)* [PDF file]. Retrieved from Quality Improvement Organization website:https://qioprogram.org/ sites/default/files/editors/141/Change_Packages_Crosswalk_20190221 _FNL_508.pdf.

Theurer, K., Mortenson, W. B., Stone, R., Suto, M., Timonen, V., & Rozanova, J. (2015). The need for a social revolution in residential care. *Journal of aging studies,* 35, 201-210.

Tierney, S., Bivins, R., & Seers, K. (2019). Compassion in nursing: Solution or stereotype? *Nursing inquiry,* 26(1), e12271.

Van Eenoo, L., van der Roest, H., Onder, G., Finne-Soveri, H., Garms-Homolova, V., Jonsson, P. V., Declercq, A. (2018). Organizational home care models across Europe: A cross sectional study. *International journal of nursing studies,* 77, 39-45.

Van Leeuwen, K. M., Van Loon, M. S., Van Nes, F. A., Bosmans, J. E., De Vet, H. C., Ket, J. C., Ostelo, R. W. (2019). What does quality of life mean to older adults? A thematic synthesis. *PLoS One,* 14(3), e0213263.

Von Dietze, E., & Orb, A. (2000). Compassionate care: a moral dimension of nursing. *Nursing Inquiry,* 7(3), 166-174.

West, M., Eckert, R., Collins, B., & Chowla, R. (2017). *Caring to change: how compassionate leadership can stimulate innovation in health care*. London: The King's Fund.

White, H. K., Corazzini, K., Twersky, J., Buhr, G., McConnell, E., Weiner, M., & Colón-Emeric, C. S. (2012). Prioritizing culture change in nursing homes: Perspectives of residents, staff, and family members. *Journal of the American Geriatrics Society,* 60(3), 525-531.

Young, A., & Tinker, A. (2017). *The 1960s baby boomers: future needs and preferences*. Working with Older People.

Zimmerman, S., & Cohen, L. W. (2010). Evidence behind The Green House and similar models of nursing home care. *Aging Health*, 6(6), 717-737.

Zimmerman, S., Shier, V., & Saliba, D. (2014). Transforming nursing home culture: Evidence for practice and policy. *Gerontologist,* 54(Suppl_1), S1-S5.

In: Elderly Care
Editor: Sean M. Eckstein

ISBN: 978-1-53618-446-4

Chapter 4

ELDERLY HOMES AND ELDERLY CARE IN LEBANON

Ramzi Nasser[1,*] ***and Jacqueline Doumit***[2]
Education Department, University of Sharjah, Sharjah, UAE
Department of Nursing & Health Sciences, Notre Dame University, Zouk Mosbeh, Lebanon

ABSTRACT

Lebanon is an Arabic speaking country located further east of the Mediterranean Sea. Elderly in Lebanon has reached 11.1% of the population 6.85 million. The Lebanese population demographics have changed over the two decades with immigration of the young to outside the country and consequently older age population has greatly burdened the health care system. Little is known about elderly homes and services provided for the elderly residing in these Lebanese long term care institutions. While the country brandishes itself as leading in health and medical services in the Middle East region, there is still a shortage of health care providers/professionals who are specialized in geriatrics. Even with the very aging population and the growing number of long term care

* Corresponding Author's Email: ramzinaimnasser@hotmail.com.

institutions, elderly homes (mostly private) face challenges in support facilities, standard accreditation, professional staffing, oversight to its health services, management, human resources, accreditation, nutritional status and infrastructure capacities. This study/chapter will report the status of elderly homes in Lebanon, including socio-demographic changes, social and economic developments, health services and financing. Lebanon like other developing countries is in need to improve standards, practices and policies, and to enforce their implementations in order to improve the quality of life among elderly home dwellers. There is also a need to ensure the availability of health and social services for older persons and promote their continuing participation in social and productive life. The chapter will provide further discussions and recommendations in the health sector for elderly home dwellers in Lebanon.

Keywords: elderly, elderly homes, accreditation, quality, population

INTRODUCTION

Lebanon, or the Lebanese Republic, is a small country (4,036 square mile) in the East Mediterranean. The population of Lebanon is estimated at 6.86 million in 2019, up from the 4.43 million in 2013 (Lebanon Population, 2019). There has been a surge in the population due to the current flux of refugees escaping war in neighboring Syria. Census in Lebanon has not been taken since 1930s and not seen since the inception of the republic (Maktabi, 1999). Currently, Lebanon is also one of the densest in the world and has 1507 people per square mile (Lebanon Population, 2019). With the refugees return to Syria and the constant migration of Lebanese people, the expectation is that the population will start to decline around 2025 (Lebanon Population, 2019) and will projected to reach 4,701,000 by 2030 (Sibai, Rizk and Kronfol, 2017).

The population of elderly (65 years old and above) was about 428,811 in 2017 (World Health Organization, 2017) and the life expectancy among elderly was about 80.27 years for males and 82.11 years for females (El-Khoury, Kosremelli-Asmar, and Stephan-Yeretzian, 2012). Moreover, the percentage of elderly predicted in Sibai, Sen, Baydoun and Saxen (2004) study, may reach 10.25% of the population by 2025 and will exceed 20% of the population by 2050 (Sibai, Rizk and Kronfol, 2017).

The increase in the proportion of the elderly (60 years old and above) in Lebanon has reached 11.1% in 2006 (Ministry of Public Health, 2007). A relatively high percentage of Lebanese older people (close to 99%) live alone (Doumit, Nasser and Bitar, 2010) which is similar to that seen in some Western nations (Sibai, Rizk and Kronfol, 2017) and is one of the highest rates among neighboring Arab nations (United Nations Population Fund, 2017). The growth of elderly in proportion and absolute level has raised some alarm in the developed world; while somewhat downplayed in the developing world in the assumption that the family has a strong sense of collective and extended families will take care of the aging population (Hamade, Ghobeira and Yassin, n.d.).

Society in Lebanon is close-knit and elderly care has been predominantly family-based. With the immigration of young adult especially after the flare of last regional conflict with Israel in 2006, the ever shrinking nuclear family, and the greater number of women in the workforce, elderly are more likely to live alone, isolated, in custodial setting and are more likely to face health related issues (Nasser and Doumit, 2011).

The demographic of elderly suggests also that elderly are mostly likely to be women (widows) (Doumit, Nasser and Hanna, 2014; Doumit and Nasser, 2010) and up to 82% of poor women come from households where the husband has been the sole breadwinner; they have no pension plan and are left to their own devices (Hamade, Ghobeira and Yassin, n.d.). A 2004 survey of living conditions indicated that approximately a quarter of Lebanese households and 38.4% of the elderly live in poverty and less likely to afford the support they need in elderly homes (Abou Shawarab, Houri, Naja, 2010).

Economic and Social Change and Its Impact on Health

In Lebanon, the traditional role of the family in caring for the elderly has declined in the past two decades. The role of family members towards the elderly has been influenced by work commitments of all the family members and the complexities of everyday life that have negatively impacted elderly lives particularly losing their social status, esteem and respect (Abou Shawarab, Haouri, and Naja, 2010). In some cases, the elderly face isolation, lack of fiscal independence, loss of social interaction and distance from family members (Abou Shawarab, Haouri, and Naja, 2010). It also reflects an increase in the number of young Lebanese immigrants especially young women who mostly likely to offer the caring role for the elderly in the family (Abou Shawarab, Haouri, and Naja, 2010). With the dire economic situation in Lebanon, it appears that the situation is difficult for low-income families particularly for elderlies who are unable to secure expenses of basic living with the absence of the extended family and family nets (Abou Shawarab, Haouri, and Naja, 201). Moreover, 53.3% of the elderly population residing in Lebanon does not benefit from any health insurance, even with the increase of dependency ratio (defined as the number of persons aged 65 years and above per 100 persons between the ages of 15 to 64), topped by an increase in elderly disabilities which is estimated to be 27.3% (Abou Shawarab, Houri, Naja, 2010).

Over the past few decades, the changes of lifestyle including increased tobacco consumption, reduced physical activity and unbalanced dietary intake accompanied with unplanned urbanization, Lebanon had a significant negative impact on the health of the elderly (Sibai, Rizk and Kronfol, 2014). The dominant infectious diseases are being replaced by chronic non-communicable diseases (NCDs), being the major causes of death (Sibai, Rizk and Kronfol, 2014). It is estimated that, near 50% of the Eastern Mediterranean region's burden of disease is due to NCDs (Khatib, 2004). Particularly, the region has been identified as having highest rates of diabetes in the world and one of the highest comparative prevalence of diabetes worldwide (over 20% among older people worldwide). In addition, Lebanon shows a high level of hypertension (up to 50%) and alarming levels of obesity (around 40%). Another disabling factor which accounts to 50% of death in older adults is the prevalence of cardiovascular diseases and stroke which are rapidly growing and represent the main underlying causes of morbidity and death, notably among older persons (Sibai, Fletcher, Hills and Campbell, 2001). Cancer is another major leading cause of death in Arab countries. In Lebanon, almost 15% of mortalities are due to cancer (Yount and Sibai, 2009).

Table 1. The composition of elderly population as of 2017

Age Range	Population		Deaths		Epidemiology		
	Female (N)	Male (N)	Female (%)	Male (%)	Diabetes Mellitus* (N)	Cardiovascular diseases* (N)	Neoplasms (N)
65-69	75,152	77,310	2.99	4.73	812	5,394	2,542
70-74	61,890	61,890	4.2	5.37	671	4,735	2,025
75-79	39,786	44,207	5.4	6.51	570	4,854	1,475
80-84	26,524	26,524	6.65	7.12	352	3,701	859
85+	8,841	13,262	11.07	9.6	242	3,412	510
Total	212,193	223,193	30.31	33.37	2,647	22,096	7,411

* By the Ministry of Public Health (2007).

While NCDs are becoming common, depression is also a common psychiatric problem among older adults in the Middle East region and deementia taking its toll among older adults and possible reasons to why elderly are being placed in custodial settings (i.e., elderly homes) by guardians (Sibai, Rizk, and Kronfol, 2014).

Elderly Homes

Elderly homes in Lebanon date back to the beginning of the twentieth century, where they had a limited role to shelter displaced elderly providing boarding, hostel services, food, and limited medical services (Abou Shawarab, Haouri, and Naja, 2010). By the middle of the twentieth century, religious and charitable establishments took the initiative to establish and provide care for the elderly through nursing and day-to-day social services (Abou Shawarab, Haouri, and Naja, 2010).

Currenlty several types of institutions offer services to elderly, these include; elderly homes or long term care institutions which have increased in number from 33 in 2005 to 46 in 2008. They comprised approximately

4,100 beds and 3,299 elderly people, equivalent to 0.8% of the total elderly population in Lebanon, compared to 3,670 beds and 2,106 elderly in 2005 (Doumit, Nasser, Bitar 2010). Currently, there are approximately 49 long term care institutions with more than 4,000 beds and some of them include rehabilitation centers and older adult centers (Abou Shawarab, Haouri, and Naja, 2010); second, day institutions (n=58) which include elderly day clubs offering day services as food and shelter; and third, home services (n=74) including clinics and restaurants (Abou Shawarab, Haouri, and Naja, 2010). The number of beds or the number of institutions has increased to meet the growing demand. Many of the institutions are within proximity to the suburbs, are crowded and have a long waiting list for elderly to seek admission. On the other hand, the elderly homes in rural areas have vacant beds (Abou Shawarab, Haouri, and Naja, 2010; Doumit and Nasser, 2010). In the capital Beirut and its surrounding as of 2017 there are a critical mass of 412,512 elderly which comes to about 50% of the elderly population (World Health Organization, 2017). The critical mass of elderly homes are located in or around the two major cities in Lebanon being greater Beirut and Tripoli (Doumit and Nasser 2010). The demand for elderly homes outweighs the capacity of elderly homes (Abou Shawarab, Haouri, and Naja, 2010).

Elderly homes or long-term care institutions that care or provide services for the elderly are spread over all Lebanese governed areas (i.e., states). The majority are concentrated in the Mount Lebanon region with 28 institutions (61%), followed by 10 in the North (23%), 7 in Beirut (7%), 3 in Bekaa (Eastern part of Lebanon) (7%), and 1 in the South (2%) (Abou Shawarab, Haouri, and Naja, 2010). The number of beds, in elderly homes are distributed as follows: 15 institutions (42%) with no more than 50 beds, 14 institutions (39%) with 50 to 100 beds, and 6 institutions (17%) with more than 100 beds. The majority of institutions belong to private-charitable, religious, or civil associations (Doumit and Nasser, 2010). The cities and their suburbs hold the majority of able populace which are employed and have no one at home to support the elderly. Conversely in rural areas, close-knit family structures allow for elderly care to be provided at home (Doumit and Nasser, 2010).

Many elderly homes in Lebanon provide services, not limited to include housing, social care but also palliative care and end of life care (Abou Shawarab, Houri, Naja, 2010). Other elderly homes or skilled nursing facilities receive incapacitated elderly either with physical or at mental disabilities. They treat elderly with various illnesses and diseases; having limited professioal capacity, they provide services mostly human to support the elderly (Abou Shawarab, Houri, Naja, 2010). Many of these elderly homes do not separate between independent and dependent elderly who are mentally incapacitated (Doumit and Nasser, 2010).

Residents in long term nursing or elderly homes develop strong social relationships with home care personnel or caregivers that require a unique approach to the interpersonal aspects of nursing. It has been found that the nurse-patient interaction is a vital resource for promoting physical, emotional, functional, social and spiritual well-being among nursing home patients (Haugan, Hanssen, and Moksnes, 2013). Many of the elderly may suffer from low self-esteem, lack a sense of personal worth, lack the ability to control of their personal life, and lack confidence and hope. They need the social support and care from people around them who are able to understand their feelings, and their psychological and social needs. The shortage of specialized staff has led institutions, to resort to hire foreign labor with lower pay-scale, and most likely resulting in the inability of the elderly to communicate with the carer to meet their needs. By putting foreign caregivers, elderly will more likely withdraw, to become alienated, or to fall into depression (Doumit and Nasser, 2010).

Many of the elderly homes may employ medical or professional elderly care staff. However, elderly do rarely interact with geriatric medical professionals (Abou Shawarab, Houri, and Naja, 2010). Current statistics show that 30.6% of 49 elderly homes lack the needed social workers and social practitioners to support elderly and reintegrate them in society (Abou Shawarab, Houri, and Naja, 2010). Moreover, there is a serious lack of geriatricians; approximately there is one geriatric doctor for every 20,000 persons aged 65 or over (Sibai, Rizk, and Kronfol, 2014). In addition, the level of care differs from one elderly home to another and the ratio of elderly to caregivers is not well understood. The majority of staff in nursing homes work 12 hours a day for 6 days a week at the minimum or low wage (Doumit, Nasser and Bitar 2010). The health workers engagement with the elderly often stems from the reality of the job and the associated wages (Doumit, Nasser and Bitar, 2010). There is no career path or association for caregiver professional to draw them into the labor force and to register them in the National Social Security Fund (NSSF). It is noteworthy to mention that training in geriatric care exists in higher education institutions; Lebanon offers a gerontology program for nurses and geriatric courses to medical students. Although there are specialized program for medical physicians terminating in a diploma in geriatrics or gerontology, still however, there is a great demand for geriatrics in the field. Actually, the number of geriatricians doubled from 8 in 2008 (Sibai et al., 2011) and the expectation might reach to about 16 in 2020.

FUNDING

Lebanon was under the French mandate after World War I and in 1943 the Ministry of Public Relief was created. The NSSF within the Ministry of Public Relief was established in 1964 as a model of the French system which included funds for retirement as end-of-service pension, maternity and sickness. The NSSF adopted the fee-for-service model, in which patients receive care and then are reimbursed by the NSSF. The care is generally provided by a network of providers registered with the NSSF. Those included private hospitals and community ones. With the onset of the civil war which started in the 1970s and continued throughout the 1980s, the NSSF got derailed and operated in a dysfunctional manner, it mainly served those public servants as the military, security and government employees. As of the 1990s the elderly were not given any sort of health insurance. Public employees can choose between a retirement pension and an indemnity of retirement; if they choose indemnity they generally receive a lump sum payment equal to one month of each year they were employed in, two months if they worked for ten to thirty years and three months for more than thirty years. Employees in the private sector, covered by the NSSF during their productive years, are deprived of the health insurance coverage on retirement from work at 64 years old leaving the elderly with no substantial support once they reach the old age.

Overall, public servants enjoy better insurance coverage and benefits than those in the private sector with wide variations in the level of basic benefits for retirees and inequitable coverage by sector of employment. Otherwise the elderly tend to pick their own private insurance with exuberant fees; many elderly who apply to subscribe at later age are disqualified practically because of their age and the possible onset of disease.

Lebanon is one of the few countries that provides a lump-sum pension for employees of the private sector. The government does little in managing the pension plan. Elderly, who may seek to support themselves in managing those funds, find themselves completely isolated. Their very low levels of educational attainment, dwindling economic capacity, absence of a pension plans, and limited workforce participation fuels their ability to sustain themselves financialy which among the poorly educated is harder than expected of them to survive. Among older women, the situation is particularly precarious. Moreover, the prevalent poverty status deprived them of adequate access to quality health services, water, electricity and housing. A study by Sibai, Ghanem and Wall (2007) suggest that after the July 2006-War on Lebanon, the study concluded that in comparison to other population segments, the elderly appeared to be the most fiscally vulnerable population having higher difficulty in maintaining and attaining their basic needs.

Care for the elderly has significant ramification on the ability of elderly to pay for their care. Many of the self-employed as those in the informal sector, and an estimate of only 24.1% of women in the Middle East and North Africa region aged 15-64 are legally part of the labor force (Sibai, Rizk, and Kronfol, 2014). In Lebanon, in particular, there is a gray economy where 42% to 55% of agricultural employees and other family-type business are informally employed in unregistered small enterprises and family businesses which do not contribute to the pension schemes (Robalino et al., 2005) and thus are less likely to contribute to the qualify for old-age pension plans and thus make contribution they make into the pension system. Lebanon has issued the 'optional' health insurance scheme for the elderly, but it was frozen in 2006. It could be estimated that social security coverage extends to less than 25% of the population in Lebanon and the Arab region, the reason for the low coverage is because of the labor market, predominance of the gray market or land labor-agricultural trade which is not completely regulated by government. Thus, elderly rely predominantly on the savings, informal support and through charitable organizations.

The sources of funding for elderly homes comes mainly from private and personal funding. However, some elderly homes are registered as community centers and for non-profit while the Ministry of Public Health does not contact elderly homes to provide the health care needed as in a contractor or purchaser but it provides in-kind resources to a network of primary care (medical and public health services). The government for instance provides in-kind monies: 36% are contracted with the Ministry of Public Health, 44% contracted with the Ministry of Social Affairs, and 44% receive special assistance. Doumit, Nasser, and Bitar (2010) revealed that the monthly amounts paid to institutions by elderly ranged from 50,000 to 2,250,000 Lebanese pounds, which comes to about a respective range from 33 to 1500 US Dollars. The Ministry of Public Health, provides each elderly resident in these institutions an amount of 15,600 Lebanese pounds per day, which comes to about 10 US Dollars; while the Ministry of Social Affairs contributes an amount of 4,100 Lebanese pounds per day for each elderly person which comes to an amount of 1.33 US Dollars (Nasser and Doumit, 2011). The expenses of elderly-stay are offset through private funding for those without financial resources or unable to pay the expenses of their elderly homes. It is reported that about 20% of elderly homes medicine costs are generally divided equally between the elderly own funds and the elderly homes. Concomitantly 60% of the elderly homes provide the medicine and other medical services and procedures.

Many of the community-based, non-profit institutions are affiliated to the religious and/or sectarian organizations and generally bare the costs of elderly through philanthropy. The elderly homes have also the affiliation, funding and organization established by sectarian entities. Still however, the elderly struggle with the payments and support at homes. Lebanon still relies heavily on a non-formal social system especially the family or community-based social support. This formal neglect i.e., government social policy is based on the male-breadwinner model of family structure which prioritizes the economic activity of the man/father (patriarchal structure); within this overarching framework and long-term care needs of older persons it tends to be seen and dominated by a patriarchal system where older women are seen to be the most vulnerable segement in society to receive elderly home-care.

CULTURAL AND SOCIAL ISSUES

In many cultures as well as the Middle East, family network is very strong and tight. The family structure is generally hierarchical with the elderly sitting at the top of the hierarchy as a source of knowledge, guidance, wisdom, a binding figure and often providing moral and religious guidance. The family in its extensions (extended family) draws on the group for support and safety and assumes the responsibility for those in need. Also the Lebanese cultural pattern is collectivist that people are focused on relationships and connections with others, rather than achievements of the individual; they are more disposed to humility and collective will (Heine, et al., 1999). Accordingly, the family often assumes responsibility for the welfare of the elderly by helping in daily chores, and providing financial and social support. Typically, those carers at home are middle-aged married daughters, who look after an older impaired relative, particularly those with memory loss (Séoud et al., 2007; Abou Shawarab, Houri, Naja, 2010). Long-term care is a physically and mentally arduous responsibility and it is not unusual, for caregivers to incur health problems themselves. While such customs and traditions persist today predominantly in rural areas, it is now almost impossible to maintain this social structure. With the onset of the civil war back in 1975, the deterioration of the economic and the large immigration of the youth, it was proving impossible that such network remains knitted to support its extensions and mainly the elderly. While the social structure is reflected in all sectarian groups, Christians, Druze and Muslims, there are little differences in the approach of elderly among the three main sects (Abyad, 2001). The new sprouting of elderly homes has come with the greater demand for rooms and elderly services in their homes, as extended family being scattered or because of fiscal circumstances, many of the families are now reaching to outsource the care for the elderly, they may have no other alternative as those who are healthy and need little physical support may find it difficult to find the social and psychological support needed. They rely on extended line of friendships and relations in the collective. The replacement of the family has also been taken over by non-governmental/non-profit agencies, with smaller families, and traditional patterns of family responsibility diminishing with economic development traditional patterns of care will also diminish. With increased urbanization, young city dwellers will have difficulty taking care of their elderly, coupled with intense migration and the high cost of living makes it too difficult for the young to integrate the elderly in their lives. This problem will remain and the need for elderly homes with quality care is no less significant than providing financial health insurance for the elderly. More so the need to hear the voices of elderly and needs and address them "has never been heard as loud."

ACCREDITATION

Since mid-2000 a quality assurance control and process was imputed in Lebanon where hospitals and care centers started to implement standards of practice, gradually shifting from structures, safety and equipment to processes, clinical outcomes, quality care, and policies. Many of the elderly homes run as hospital providers are keen about the quality services, quality assurance and improvement- many homes are in the process of enumerating established organizational structures, regular meetings, maintainance of patient records, files and follow-up, improvements, alignments to established standards and good practices.

The Ministry of Public Health played a major role in the development of the criteria and accreditation, it has developed an external evaluation system for hospitals with the declared aim of promoting continuous quality improvement. This was possible through shere pragmatisim in interpretating of an existing law, without the need for a new legislation (approval by the ministerial council and approval by the Ministry of Public Health). The Ministry sought international expertise to overcome allegations of partiality, and the accreditation was intentionally presented as an activity independent of the Government and other stakeholders to foster elements of oversight and transparency (Accreditation Standards for Hospitals, 2019).

Accreditation standards were developed following a consensus building process. Hospitals were audited against these standards in a professional, educative, non-threatening manner and confidential manner. Results from the first round audit revealed a shocking failure by majority of hospitals in complying with basic standards, only to recover through follow-up, re-audit, showing a better use of resources and a higher degree of commitment to their mission and objectives. This allowed for the revisions of the standard criteria and another round of auditing. The step-wise approach adopted by the Ministry ensured a smooth and gradual elderly home involvement, and led to the creation of a shift towards quality practices. The Ministry of Public Health's 's undeclared aim was in fact to strengthen its regulative capabilities and attain better value for money in terms of government investment and hospital care financing. As the selection of hospitals to be contracted could then be made on objective quality criteria, freeing the system from any kind of favoritism or discrimination, especially confessional and political ones (Accreditation Standards for Hospitals, 2019).

Nutritional Status of Elderly

Malnutrition is frequent among elderly living in long-term care institutions (Donini et al., 2013; Vandewoude and Van Gossum, 2013). Its impact is empirically established with reports of increased mortality

(Söderström, Rosenblad, Adolfsson, Saletti, and Bergkvist, 2014), increased morbidity (Correia and Waitzberg, 2003) and increased elderly health-care costs (Abbasi and Rudman, 1994). Malnutrition is also associated with several health risk factors, among them are functional activity (Mamhidir et al., 2006; Romero-Ortuno et al., 2011; Stange, Poeschl, Stehle, Sieber, and Volkert, 2013), psycho-cognitive (Rodriguez-Tadeo et al., 2012), oral health problems (De Marchi et al., 2008) and comorbidities (Chavarro-Carvajal et al., 2015). The improvement of socio-economic, oral, functional and psychological health conditions may improve the nutritional status and the quality of life among the elderly, whether in home care or living free.

In Lebanon, a national study conducted on elderly residing in 36 nursing homes distributed in all regions found that the majority of residents had low socio-economic status and poor health. The prevalence of malnutrition and the risk of malnutrition were 3.2% and 27.6% respectively with no statistically significant difference between women and men on Mini Nutritional Assessment and body mass index (Doumit, Nasser, and Hanna, 2014). Moreover, a high percentage of elderly (reaching 100 percent) had a low intake of energy, protein, linolenic acid, linoleic acid, fibers, vitamins and minerals, and the prevalence of nutrient inadequacy was significantly different between sexes for copper intake (Doumit and Nasser, 2017). In addition, three studies examined the nutritional status and associated risk factors among Lebanese elderly residing in nursing homes (El Zoghbi et al., 2013; Sibai, Zard, Adra, Baydoun, and Hwalla, 2003; Doumit, 2015). The first study covered a single urban area, the capital Beirut, and a small number of institutions (El-Zoghbi et al., 2013), they compared the nutritional status between institutionalized residing in 4 nursing homes and non-institutionalized elderly and found that elderly residents consumed more fat and fibers, were anemic, had low levels of albumin and suffered from several minerals and vitamins deficiencies including zinc, magnesium, α-tocopherol, vitamin A and D, and pyridoxine (Sibai, Zard, Adra, Baydoun & Hwalla, 2003). The second study conducted by El-Zoghbi et al., 2013 observed that 12.6% of elderly residing in three nursing homes were malnourished and 48.7% were at risk of malnutrition. Moreover, a high percentage (71.43%) of malnourished residents showed a cognitive function deterioration (El-Zoghbi et al., 2013). Lastly, Doumit's (2015) study indicated that factors related to nutritional intake, was functional impairment followed by oral health problems and depression. In general, there are high levels of malnourishment found among unemployed elderly who had no jobs and had oral health problems, functional impairment and depression.

FUTURE DIRECTIONS

Certainly a long-term strategy is needed for the development of elderly care in Lebanon. The creation of the National Permanent Commission for the Care of Senior Citizens Affairs, has established a number of day-care institutions for the elderly known as clubs, also the initiative to start accreditation process as a continuous quality assurance process (Accreditation Standards for Hospitals, 2019). Other initiatives devised by the Ministry of Public Health its 20-year strategy in the development of a community-based care system where primary care resources are situated in the community that assist the family in its traditional role of supporting the elderly in their homes through home visitations and support. Care of patients needs are then shared by family members and professional services. Certainly, Lebanon can take advantage of the rich cultural and societal and family values and social practices. Seemly the role of the family and the intergenerational support system in the care of older relatives, can engage the informal caregivers as a resource and as beneficiaries of care. Hence, greater emphasis needs to be placed on the creation policies that link elderly pension with home stay support initiatives. Accepting long-term care services as the last recourse when all community alternative is exhausted.

Further, Lebanon is in dire need to establish a new pension plan targeting old-age income security systems feature poverty reduction strategies and aim at providing some form of basic income security to all persons in old age. Pension systems could include poor elderly who have not contributed to the NSSF and offering minimum benefits financed by taxation or cooperate awareness schemes as in giving back to society. Corporation and private establishments need to rethink their contribution to government and protect its employees after retirement.

Further, preemptive measures of health awareness and elderly health systems may lead to early prevention may significantly lead a better later life for the elderly. Making healthier choices at an early stage may impact later life health choices. It also draws on those aspects of early intervention through health promotion awareness- disease prevention and early screening. Thus, community centers and clinics may provide early screening, health educational material and follow-up feedback. Virtual social network and technology can play a significant role in keeping elderly updated on good nutrition and advanced lifelong health promotions. Further, Lebanon and other Arab countries homes and public spaces or even home utilities could function to provide places for the elderly to engage and carry out their daily activities. More so, hospitals and care centers need to assess not only the quality of care but also the elderly conditions with immediate and on-sight diagnostic whether in psychological or nutritional intake.

While the discourse of the elderly wellbeing support comes from the view of the elderly in terms of the welfare concept of support. Elderly ability to become empowered reflects the aspirations and rights to be independent and choose their living. A focus on human rights paradigm that allows for elderly autonomy, decisions, independence and daily activity is tantamount on the service culture and health system provisions. Finally, human rights embrace the rights to financial security, health and social care and safe environments. Laws for older people need to be legislated through the prism of 'human rights' and the State's obligations to its citizens, rather than through the prevalent 'welfare' optic. A focus on the human rights paradigm for advocating and implementing ageing policies can be facilitated by involving non-profit organizations and civil society particularly in societies where there are challenges found in process of engaging others in decision making. Furthermore, international human rights instruments that tackle ageism and age-based discrimination in all aspects of life need to be adopted and adapted at the national level.

ACKNOWLEDGMENT

We are grateful for the comments and suggestions on this chapter made by Dr. Nazem Bassil.

REFERENCES

Abbasi, A. and Rudman, D. (1994). Undernutrition in the nursing home: prevalence, consequences, causes and prevention, *Nutrition Reviews, 52*(4): 113-122. https://doi.org/10.1111/j.1753-4887.1994.tb01403.x.

Abou Shawarab, M., Haouri, A., and Naja, N. (2010). *National Report on Elderly Survices in Lebanon.* Population and Development Program - United Nations Population Fund - Family Affairs Department of the Ministry of Social Affairs, Beirut, Lebanon.

Abyad, A. (2001). Health care for older persons: A country profile - Lebanon. *Journal of the American Geriatrics Society, 49*(10): 1366-1370. https://doi.org/10.1046/j.1532-5415.2001.49268.x.

Accreditation Standards for Hospitals (2019). *Ministry of Public Health.* Beirut, Lebanon.

Chavarro-Carvajal, D., Reyes-Ortiz, C., Samper-Ternent, R., Arciniegas, A.J. and Gutierrez, C.C. (2015). Nutritional assessment and factors associated to malnutrition in older adults: a cross-sectional study in Bogota, Colombia, *Journal of Aging Health, 27*(2): 304-319. https://doi.org/10.1177/0898264314549661.

Correia, M.I. and Waitzberg, D.L. (2003). The impact of malnutrition on morbidity, mortality, length of hospital stay and costs evaluated through a multivariate model analysis, *Clinical Nutrition, 22*(3): 235-239. https://doi.org/10.1016/S0261-5614(02)00215-7.

De Marchi, R.J., Hugo, F.N., Hilgert, J.B. and Padilha, D.M. (2008). Association between oral health status and nutritional status in south Brazilian independent-living older people, *Nutrition, 24*(6): 546-553. https://doi.org/10.1016/j.nut.2008.01.054.

Donini, L. M., Scardella, P., Piombo, L., Neri, B., Asprino, R., Proietti, A. R., Carcaterra, S., Cava, E., Cataldi, S., Cucinotta, D., Di Bella, G., Barbagallo, M., and Morrone, A. (2013). Malnutrition in elderly: Social and economic determinants. *Journal of Nutritional Health Aging, 17*(1): 9–15. https://doi.org/10.1007/s12603-012-0374-8.

Doumit J. (2015). Malnutrition and associated risk factors among elderly living in Lebanese community homes. *Nutrition and Food Science, 45*(3): http://dx.doi.org/10.1108/NFS-09-2014-0084.

Doumit, J. and Nasser, R. (2010). Quality of life and wellbeing of the elderly in Lebanese nursing homes, *International Journal of Health Care Quality Assurance, 23*(1): 72-93. https://doi.org/10.1108/09526861011010695.

Doumit, J. and Nasser, R. (2017). Nutrients intake in elderly residing in Lebanese nursing homes, *Nutrition and Food Science, 47*(2): 217-228. https://doi.org/10.1108/NFS-06-2016-0070.

Doumit J., Nasser R. and Bitar C. (2010). Reality and challenges of the elderly nursing homes in Lebanon. *Human and Health Magazine*. 10,7-9 (in Arabic).

Doumit, J. H., Nasser, R. N., and Hanna, D. R. (2014). Nutritional and health status among nursing home residents in Lebanon: comparison across gender in a national cross sectional study. *BMC Public Health, 14*(1): 629. doi: 10.1186/1471-2458-14-629.

El-Khoury, W., Kosremelli-Asmar, M., and Stephan-Yeretzian, J. (2012). *National health statistics report in Lebanon*, Institute of Health Management and Social Protection, 58-62.

El-Zoghbi, M., Boulos, C., Al Hajje, A., Saleh, N., Awada, S., Rachidi, S., Bawab, W. and Salameh, P. (2013). Associations between cognitive function and nutritional status in elderly: a cross-sectional study in three institutions of Beirut – Lebanon, *Geriatric Mental Health Care, 1*(4): 73-81. https://doi.org/10.1016/j.gmhc.2013.04.007.

Hamade, A. S. H., Ghobeira, M. G., and Yassin, N. (n.d.) *Assessing the Lebanese Elderly welfare pension reform: Time for a new policy*. Amerian University of Beirut.

Haugan, G., Hanssen B., and Moksnes U., K. (2013). Self-transcendence, nurse-patient interaction and the outcome of multidimensional well-being in cognitively intact nursing home patients. *Scand J Caring Sci. 27*(4): 882–93. https://doi.org/10.1111/scs.12000.

Heine, S. J., Lehman, D. R., Markus, H. R., and Kitayama, S. (1999). Is there a universal need for positive self-regard? *Psychological Review, 106*(4): 766-794. doi: 10.1037/0033-295X.106.4.766.

Khatib, O. (2004). Noncommunicable diseases: risk factors and regional strategies for prevention and care. *EMHJ - Eastern Mediterranean Health Journal, 10* (6): 778-788. https://apps.who.int/iris/handle/10665/119479.

Lebanon Population (2019). *World Population Review*. Accessed on 10. 20. 2019 http://worldpopulationreview.com/countries/lebanon-population/

Maktabi, R. (1999). The Lebanese census of 1932 revisited. Who are the Lebanese?. *British Journal of Middle Eastern Studies,* 26(2): 219-241.

Mamhidir, A. G., Ljunggren, G., Kihlgren, M., Kihlgren, A. and Wimo, A. (2006). Underweight, weight loss and related risk factors among older adults in sheltered housing-a Swedish follow-up study, *Journal of Nutrition Health Aging*, 10 (4): 255-262.

Ministry of Public Health (2007). *Statistical bulletin*, Beirut Lebanon.

Nasser, R. and Doumit, J. (2011). Developing criteria for Elderly nursing homes: the case of Lebanon. *Int. J Health Care Quality Assurance,* 24(3): 211-222. https://doi.org/10.1108/09526861111116651.

Robalino, D., Whitehouse, E., Mataoanu, A., Musalem, A., Sherwood, E. and Sluchynsky, O. (2005). Pensions in the Middle East and North Africa: time for change. *MPRA Paper No. 10448, Munich Personal RePEc Archive.*

Rodriguez-Tadeo, A., Wall-Medrano, A., Gaytan-Vidana, M.E., Campos, A., Ornelas-Contreras, M. and Novelo-Huerta, H.I. (2012). Malnutrition risk factors among the elderly from the US-Mexico border: the 'one thousand' study, *Journal of Nutrition Health Aging, 16*(5): 426-431. https://doi.org/10.1007/s12603-011-0349-1.

Romero-Ortuno, R., Casey, A. M., Cunningham, C. U., Squires, S., Prendergast, D., Kenny, R. A., and Lawlor, B. A. (2011). Psychosocial and functional correlates of nutrition among community-dwelling older adults in Ireland. *The Journal of Nutrition, Health & Aging, 15*(7): 527-531. https://doi.org/10.1007/s12603-010-0278-4.

Séoud, J., Nehmé, C., Atallah, R., Zablit, C., Yérétzian, J., Lévesque, L., ... and Ducharme, F. (2007). The health of family caregivers of older impaired persons in Lebanon: an interview survey. *International Journal of Nursing Studies, 44*(2): 259-272. https://doi.org/10.1016/j.ijnurstu.2005.11.034.

Sibai, A. M., Fletcher, A., Hills, M., and Campbell, O. (2001). Non-communicable disease mortality rates using the verbal autopsy in a cohort of middle aged and older populations in Beirut during wartime, 1983–93. *Journal of Epidemiology & Community Health, 55*(4): 271-276. http://dx.doi.org/10.1136/jech.55.4.271.

Sibai, A.M., Ghanem, M., and Wall, E. (2007). *Assessment of the preparedness and responsiveness of Lebanese NGOs, social clubs and clinics in the provision of services to seniors in Lebanon during and after the july-2006 war* (No. leb/02/p01). Beirut, Lebanon: Lebanese Ministry of Social Affairs and United Nations Population Fund.

Sibai, A. M., Rizk, A., and Kronfol, N. M. (2014). *Ageing in the Arab region: Trends, implications and policy options.* Center for Studies on Aging (CSA), ESCWA and UNFPA. Retrieved from http://csa.org.lb/cms/assets/csa%20publications/unfpa, 20.

Sibai, A. M., Rizk, A., and Kronfol, K. M. (2017). *Ageing in the Arab region: Trends, implications and policy options.* The United Nations Population Fund.

Sibai, A., M., Sen, K., Baydoun, M. and Saxen, P. (2004). Population ageing in Lebanon: current status, future prospects and implications for policy, World Health Organization. *Bulletin of the World Health Organization; 82*(3): 219-225.

Sibai, A., Zard, C., Adra, N., Baydoun, M. and Hwalla, N (2003). Variations in nutritional status of elderly men and women according to place of residence. *Gerontology, 49*(4): 215–224. https://doi.org/10.1159/000070401.

Söderström, L., Rosenblad, A., Adolfsson, E. T., Saletti, A., and Bergkvist, L. (2014). Nutritional status predicts preterm death in older people: a prospective cohort study. *Clinical Nutrition, 33*(2): 354-359. https://doi.org/10.1016/j.clnu.2013.06.004.

Stange, I., Poeschl, K., Stehle, P., Sieber, C. C., and Volkert, D. (2013). Screening for malnutrition in nursing home residents: comparison of different risk markers and their association to functional impairment. *The Journal of Nutrition, Health & Aging, 17*(4): 357-363. https://doi.org/10.1007/s12603-013-0021-z.

United Nations Population Fund (2017). *Population ageing and policy options in the Arab Region*, Cairo Egypt: Arab States Regional Office.

Vandewoude, M., and Van Gossum, A. (2013). Nutritional screening strategy in nonagenarians: the value of the MNA-SF (mini nutritional assessment short form) in NutriAction. *The Journal of Nutrition, Health & Aging, 17*(4): 310-314. https://doi.org/10.1007/s12603-013-0033-8.

World Health Organization (2017). *Statistical Bulletin*, Beirut Lebanon.

In: Elderly Care
Editor: Sean M. Eckstein
ISBN: 978-1-53618-446-4

Chapter 5

Care Workers and Quality of Care in Nursing Homes in Canada

Zafar Mehdi[1] ***and Ramzi Nasser***[2,*]

[1]Department of Social Sciences, Dhofar Universty, Salalah, Oman

[2]Education Department, University of Sharjah, Sharjah, UAE

Abstract

The Canadian population is rapidly ageing and there is a shortage of skilled care workers such as nurses, elder carers and care assistants in Canadian nursing homes. Care services offer older people in long-term care settings, health, psychological and social support. The advancements in health care knowledge and changing health care environment, make demands on care workers to stay abreast of their knowledge and skills to meet the changing needs of care services in home care settings and residential care facilities. Although there are mandatory and volunteer continuing training programs in long-term care sectors in Canada, the effects of further training of care workers on their career advancement, work situation and quality of care in healthcare and long-term care sector were unclear. The purpose of this chapter is to examine the impact of

* Corresponding Author's Email: ramzinaimnasser@hotmail.com.

continuing training of nursing staff in Canadian nursing 'omes and its association with the quality of care of nursing home residents. Based on theoretical premises of "Lifelong Learning Theory" it is assumed that lifelong learning (further training) of care workers in health care and long-term care is likely to have positive effects on professional development, work situation and quality of patient care. The sample of this study is care workers (nurses, elder carers and care assistants) working in healthcare sector in hospitals, home care settings and long-term nursing homes. This includes care workers; nurses (n = 947), elder carers (n = 493) and care assistants (n = 1140). Data were obtained from the latest Canadian National Survey of Work and Health of Nurses (2005). The study investigated the impact of further training of care workers quality of care in nursing homes in Canada through a multiple regression analysis technique performed on the data. It was found from this study that further training of nurses has significant and positive association with career mobility of the care workers and quality of care of nursing home residents.

Keywords: elderly, elderly care workers, basic education, furhter educational training, wages, elderly wellbeing

INTRODUCTION

Caring has varying perspectives and definitions within the research literature. In general, caring means paid or unpaid work to provide care to those who are unable to care for themselves, especially sick and elderly people. Caring for the sick refers to provision of health care to a sick or ill person either at home or in a care facility such as hospital, doctor's clinic or residential care facility. Medical definition of health care is 'the maintaining and restoration of health by the treatment and prevention of disease especially by trained and licensed professionals (as in medicine, dentistry, clinical psychology, and public health) (Merriam Webster Dictionary, 2020). It is an act of taking preventative or necessary medical procedures to improve a person's well-being. It may be done with surgery in hospital or the administering of drugs or other alterations in a person's lifestyle.

Regulating caring is offered through health care systems. Health care professionals such as nurses and health workers play a crucial role in delivering health care to the sick. The education and training play a significant role in the professionalization of health workers in providing quality health care. Canada as other developed countries has well developed, regulated system for nurses and health workers in education and professional practice. This chapter looks at the education and experience of health professionals in relation to elderly-quality health variables.

Canada is experiencing demographic changes with an increasing elderly population and rising life expectancy. These demographic changes in Canada reflect the increase in paid formal care in health care and long-term care sectors. Care workers like nurses, elder carers and care assistants play a key role in the successful delivery of healthcare in nursing homes and hospitals for elderly in custodial settings which require constant health support. Care workers must continuously upgrade their professional knowledge and skills through lifelong learning to provide competent and quality of care services to elderly in nursing homes.. Continuing training of care workers can open doors to new horizons and career opportunities. Although continuing professional development in areas of expertise, through specialty courses and advanced education is essential to instill best practice approach. Since the increase in the number of elderly people, medical advancement, restructuring of health care and long-term care system and continuous changes in health care technology; demand for continuing training of skilled care workers. These changes in Canada affect health care and especially the long-term care system.

Care workers constitute a combination of regulated (nurses) and unregulated (elder carers and care assistants) care providers. They are accountable for direct or indirect care services of health care users in hospitals, long-term residential care facilities and home care settings (Canadian Nurses Association, 2015). Care workers come with different level of training and education which aligns to their employment status (Burau, Theobald and Blank, 2007). The type and amount of nursing education and training determines care workers' competency, professional development and their ability to provide quality and effective patient care. As care workers complete their basic occupational education and training, and become active members of health care or long-term care industry, their education and training does not end. They can continue to enhance their knowledge and skills by participating in additional training opportunities. In the everchanging field of health care, further training of nurses has become a requirement (Beth, 2019). Many educational programs have been initiated in long-term care facilities, but the effectiveness of additional training in long-term care is still unclear (Aylward, et al., 2003).

AGING, CARE NEEDS AND SKILLED CARE WORKERS

Since 1961, Canada has seen a decline in fertility and longevity causing a demographic change in the population. From 1980 to 2020, Canadian population 65 and older is growing at an increasing rate as a percentage of the overall population. As a consequence, changes in the proportion of older adults (aged 65 years and older) and the older adults (75 years old and over) is dramatically growing (Statistics Canada, 2016). The elderly people who have health problems are unable to, or have difficulty performing their basics of daily living; dressing, eating, getting around, toileting hygiene and so on. As this occurs, the demands for elder care support increase. Policy makers, governments and health care institutions ensure that all clients/or care services users in hospitals, long-term residential care facilities and home care settings, receive proper care and care workers who deliver direct or indirect care services to their clients, must stay current with their updated knowledge and skills of care. Why this table or boxes?

The baby boomers in Canada constitutes 29% of the population and all are expected to retire by 2029 (Statistics Canada, 2016). An analysis of today's demographics suggests that by the year 2036, 25% of the entire population will be over the age of 65 (Canadian Institute for Health Information, 2010). More than 7% of Canadians receiving long-term care services, 4.5% will be in residential care settings and 2.6% were receiving care at their homes (Statistics Canada, 2014).

Table 1 points out that the percentages of aged people; 65 and above and 80 and older in Canada. According to United Nations (1999) 100 years demographic estimates of indicators (1950-2050). With the current estimates, Canada, is in shortage of long-term elderly homes. Thee problem is not restricted to individuals waiting in hospitals; but many are waiting in their own homes for nursing home beds (C.D Howe Institute, 2013). Many are finding it difficult to live independently without informal or formal support and may require a range of services in the community, hospitals or care homes.

Table 1. The Percentage of the population age 65 and above in Canada 1980-2020

	Percentage 65 and older			Percentage 80 and older		
Country	1980	2000	2020	1980	2000	2020
Canada	9.4	12.8	18.2	1.8	3.1	4.4

Source: United Nations. Department of International Economic, United Nations. Department for Economic, Social Information, & Policy Analysis. (1999). World population prospects (Vol. 2). United Nations, Department of International, Economic and Social Affairs.

Long-Term Residential Care Facilities (Nursing Homes)

The residential care facilities are facilities with four beds or more that are funded, licensed or approved by provincial/territorial departments of health and/or social services (Statistics Canada 2014). Residential care facility for the elderly persons is a form of housing and service provision.

Long-term residential care facilities such as nursing homes or assisted living homes have become extremely important when frail elderly and older disabled people feel that it is difficult for them to continue living in their own or family homes independently. They need to find alternative care services to stay for a longer period of time. These safer places are residential care facilities where they are taken care of for 24/7 by skilled nursing staff. The residential care facilities provide secure living, personal care, assistance and support, nutritious meals, basic linen, personal laundry services, recreational and activity programs (Canadian Institute for Health

Information, 2010). The concept of residential care appeared in the 1960s as a form of institutionalized long-term care for the poor (Kane, Kane and Ladd, 1998). Other types of residential care facilities that accounts for long-term care provided to adults and children who stay in a residential setting rather than in their own home or family home. All the types of institutional structure are supported by elderly health professional who demand continuous training and retraining.

In Canada, a proportion of elderly are in the residential care i.e., elderly homes and the majority are in their homes (88%) (see Table 2 for more details) waiting time institutionalized in care homes is longer than other European countries. In 2012, there were more than 40% of alternative care (eligible for residential care) patients were waiting in acute care hospitals for residential care facilities (Canadian Institute for Health Information, 2012) and almost 59% of inpatient rehabilitation were also waiting for residential care. According to Canadian Institute for Health Information (2012), in Canada the average wait time for a bed was approximately 154 days. During this waiting time, either patients stay in hospitals and sent to their homes.

Table 2. Care Receivers and long-term care beds in different Care Settings

Long-term Care Bed						
Long-term Care receivers (%)			(Per 1000 Population aged 65 and older) %			
Year	Country	Residential care	Home care	Institutions	Hospitals	Total
2013	Canada	12.0	88.0	5.9	3.8	59.7

Sources: Statistics Canada, 2013, OECD Health Statistics 2014.

Nurses and Care Workers

Nursing is a profession within the health care sector focused on the care of individuals, families, and communities and the goal of nursing to attain, maintain, or recover optimal health and quality of life of the sick and the elderly. A medical dictionary defines 'nursing as suckling an infant as the first meaning, caring for the sick as the second, and that of the 'nurse-domestic helper' as the third, while a more general reference gives the meanings in the reverse order' (Henderson, 2006). The terms 'nurse' and 'nursing' have many meanings and have a different representation of what a nurse actually does. Definitions of nurse and nursing are understood in the perspectives of their roles they play in their nursing profession. Nurses provide care to patients, they teach and train new nurses and work in doctors' office. They have various roles across health care and long-term care settings, such as hospitals, patients' home and in residential care facilities.

Basic Educational Training in Canada

Nurses in Canada complete 12 years of high school or secondary education with a focus on the sciences, such as chemistry, physics or biology, as a requirement to be admitted to a nursing program at a professional college or nursing school in Canada (Health Force Ontario Canada, 2015). Not until 1995, the nursing profession requires a three-year diploma in a nursing program. Once prospective healthcare workers receive their qualification, they are able to register as certified nurses; however, after 1995, this requirement changed, and all provinces were encouraged to begin a four-year bachelor's degree in nursing science (Canadian Nurses Association, 2015). In Canada, all ten provinces and three territories, except Quebec, currently require a four-year bachelor's degree in nursing to practice as a registered nurse. In addition to registered nurses (RNs), there are licensed practical nurses (LPNs) and registered psychiatric nurses (RPNs), whose qualification requirements are somewhat different from those of nursing professionals.

Additional Nurse Training in Canada

Continuing or further training in nursing in Canada comes in the form of specialty courses. Registered nurses (RNs) and registered psychiatric nurses (RPNs) can undergo additional training for career development toward higher degrees. Nurses with a bachelor's degree can go through additional academic training to achieve terminal degrees such as a master's degree or a doctorate in nursing (Canadian Nurses Association, 2015).

Elder Care Training in Canada

There are various names or labels for elder carers in different provinces or professional colleges and various lengths of occupational training requirements, ranging from six to 12 months of training in elder care, to obtain a qualification in elder care (Williams, et al., 2010). Labels for elder carers include care aide, senior caregivers for elderly patients, and personal and home support workers.

Care Training and Quality of Care in Nursing Homes

Improving quality of health care is a global concern. Everyday millions of people receive high-quality health care to maintain their health. However, there are still too many people who do not get quality health care and long-term care. Quality problems are reflected in a wide variation in use of health and long-term care services and unacceptable level of medical errors in health care facilities. Improving the quality of care and reducing medical errors are priority areas of a good health care system because errors are expensive in terms of loss of trust by the client-patient leading to lower satisfaction and health services credibility (Institute of Medicine, 1999). Among the problems that commonly occur during the course of providing health care are adverse drug events, restraint-related injuries, falls, burns, pressure ulcers, and mistaken patient identities. This may be done to elderly care handling and a culture of practice in elderly and residential homes (Institute of Medicine, 1999).

McDonald et al., (2007) explained the Donabedian model of quality of health of structure, process and outcome. According to this model; structure includes the attributes of settings where care is delivered, including professional knowledge and skills of care, the process explains whether or not good medical practices are followed and outcome impacts the quality of care on health status of the clients staying at healthcare settings. In order to maintain quality of health care, appropriate and adequate care staffing with advanced skills are essential strengthen the health-care system and improves quality of care.

Quality of care is a multi-dimensional concept which has been given different meanings in research literature. For example, a client's perspective emphasizes the importance of the connection with the care they receive. One aspect of quality is seen in patients' satisfaction and is considered as a key indicator of this quality. From health care providers' perspective, the quality of the health provided by a health care can be judged by the technical performance of the care and by interpersonal relationships that occur between the health providers and customers (Mays & Pope, 2000). They further explained the technical performance as the extent to which a health care professionals provide the best practices established by medical guidelines. So when clients and patients complain, it might indicate that services are not up to par with their expectation. The World Health Organization (2006) used a number of quality statements signifying patient centered care – acceptable and taking into account preferences and aspirations of individual service users and cultures of their communities and second signifying health care which minimizes risks and harm to service users.

Research literature specifies that nurse training and further education is positively associated with patient outcomes. For example, numerous empirical studies are evident that hospitals employment of nurses with a baccalaureate level or higher degree and employed in hospitals was associated with improved patient outcomes (Linda, et al., 2003). According to Aiken et al., (2003) plentiful studies have demonstrated the relationship between higher levels of nursing education and improved patient outcomes. Aiken's et al., (2003) study also demonstrated that all else being equal, the odd of 30-day mortality and failure to rescue were reduced by 5% with every 10% increase in Bachelor Degree in Nursing. A more recent longitudinal study in 21 hospitals, Aiken et al., (2011) found that patients cared by nurses with tertiary education experienced significant reduction in length of inpatient stay, decreases in hospital acquired pressure ulcers and reduction in cardiac mortality. The value of higher levels of education has also been demonstrated in the workplace. In a survey of graduates, the National Council of State Board of Nursing (Li and Kenward, 2006) found that nurses with a tertiary education report less difficulty in managing complex patients and incorporate critical thinking in their daily practice (Li and Kenward, 2006). Empirical studies are evident that further education and training of care staff can improve patient outcomes not only in hospitals, but also in long-term care facilities (Aiken et al., (2011).

The nursing research also shows that nurses with the experience of higher education helps to reduce the nursing errors and mortality rates (Rosseter, 2012). Normally older people care is provided by a majority of licensed practical nurses (LPNs) and nurses' aides, both with less formal nursing training than Registered Nurses (RNs) especially in-home care settings (Johansson 2005). Although occupational training in the care for the elderly has only recently been recognized, still there is an increased emphasis on the need for up-skilling the workforce in health and social care (the Department of Health, London, 2007). Although few studies have emerged regarding health workers' education and training, it is imperative that education becomes pertinently linked to the workplace and best practices for quality assurance.

In Alberta, a province of Canada, researchers studied data from approximately 4800 Canadian nurses in 49 hospitals (Estabrooks et al., 2005). They found that hospitals with greater proportion of nurses educated at the level of baccalaureate level, the skill mix contained a higher proportion of registered nurses, and nurses reported good working relationships with physicians in hospitals had lower rates of mortality. In their study of 75 hospitals in Ontario, Canada, Tourangeau and colleagues (2007) found lower than a 30-day mortality rates in hospitals where nurses have had a higher level of education and a richer skill mix. Higher education in nursing is seen as a key factor in an increasingly complex and demanding care practice in hospitals in Canada (Bartels, Anke and Denise, 2012).

Data on Health Workers and Elderly and Analyses

Still few data and finding draw this relation between training of care workers on quality of patient care. We obtained data from the Canadian National Survey of Work and Health of Nurses (NSWHN, 2005). The data included 18,676 RNs, LPNs, and RPNs, who were employed in various healthcare settings in all provinces and territories of Canada. Nurses working in hospitals, long-term care facilities, and home care settings were included in this survey. Nurses answered questions on quality of patient care, including medication errors, fall injuries, and residents' complaints. We wanted to address quality issues in relation to education and training, in light of World Helath Organization quality care areas.

Different overarching regressions using two independent variables, that is, staffing level and further training. The dependent variables as quality measures of elderly health and quality measures of elderly health were the frequency of medication errors, fall injuries, complaints by older adults and nosocomial infections. A regression determined the association of further training with income, then three overarching regressions defined the predictive power of post-basic education and staffing levels on three important elder conditions. A precursor analysis using annual and employment earnings as dependent variables were regressed by the independent variables of age, post-basic training, and experience. As the years of education increase, the probability of earnings also rises. To investigate how further training affects nurses' and elder carers' annual earnings, a regression analysis was performed. The analysis evaluated the impact of further education and training to predict the quality measures of elderly health.

Elderly Health Quality Measures and Findings

Fall Injury

Table 3 presents the regression results. The analysis showed that staffing level and post-basic education had a positive association with the prevention of fall. Adequate staffing and additional nursing staff have a positive impact on prevention of fall. Adequate staffing would more likely produce 1.31 preventing residents from fall and injury. Many elderlies may need support in movement and in ways to move in elderly homes whether in daily activities or physical exercise. From the analysis of the data, it appears that the higher the training the lower the probability of injuries when there are trained staff on hand. Healthcare workers may take precaution in the way they provide greater care for older people, protecting the frail body from injury by dressing them properly and designing a safe environment. The recorded level of staffing is more significant such that the greater the number of staff members, the less likely older adults would fall. Therefore, proper staffing and training will most likely allow for pre-emptive measures to protect the latter from harm.

Table 3. Injury, medication error complaints and nosocomial infection by advanced education and staffing level

Independent variables	P-Value	Odds Ratio
Injury in a fall		
Staffing level	0.000	1.311
Post-Basic Education	0.000	1.052
Medication Error		
Staffing level	0.000	1.045
Post-Basic Education	0.000	1.015
Complaints from Patients		
Staffing level	0.000	1.240
Post-Basic Education	0.000	0.858
Nosocomial Infection		
Staffing level	0.000	1.167
Advanced Education in Nursing	0.000	1.015

Medication/Dose Errors

The second analysis investigated the association of nursing education with medication errors. The findings of the logistic regression indicated a positive association of advanced training (higher degrees) of nurses with rare medication errors (see Table 3). The odds ratio indicated that nurses with advanced training or a higher level of nursing training are 1.015 times less likely to give wrong medication to residents when compared with those with a lower level of nurse training. Adequate staffing level is also positively associated with rare medication errors. Healthcare settings with adequate staff have a 1.045 times higher probability of medication errors. Some of the functions in form of professional development and training had a positive association with preventing medication errors. Although many studies have indicated that medication errors lead to cases of morbidity and even death (Urquhart, 1994), providing on-time and correct medication improves the overall quality of care and are important elements in maintaining the health and knowledge of polypharmacy drug use among older adults. With increased staffing, there was a lesser probability of medication errors. This strong association indicates that with an appropriate staffing level, health workers can meet the required levels of care and may provide effective organizational directives.

Complaints from Residents

Canada Statistics does not measure satisfaction levels of patients to assess the quality of care, however, there are a number of variable indicators that provide an indirect measure of satisfaction, such as the number of complaints, psychological distress or a lack of daily activities in elderly home setting. The findings suggest a low probability of the number of complaints (satisfaction) associated with how health workers cared for the older adults. The health workers with an advanced level of education would have less chance to have a number of complaints. A robust generalization suggests that satisfaction with the service is strongly associated with further training of health workers. The most important influence in older adults' satisfaction is accessibility to the desired space (environment) and a health worker's continuity, humaneness, and thoroughness of care (Donabedian, 1966; Feletti, Firman, & Sanson-Fisher, 1986).

Shortage in nursing staff in busy care settings may lead to complaints from residents; accordingly, adequate staffing helps reduce the number of residents' complaints. The results showed that complaints were minimized by 1.240 times when there was adequate staff. Regarding nursing education, data showed a negative relationship between advanced nursing education and complaints. The odds ratio of 0.858 implied that nurses with advanced education were more likely to have complaint than those with a lower educational level. This finding suggests that nurses with advanced education take on several roles and responsibilities, such as administrative tasks, and thus are more likely to work with doctors, peers and sub-coordinates the whole ward and thus do not have much time to spend with all residents and their families.

Nosocomial Infection

Nosocomial infection is an avoidable infection that is more common in hospitals and it is acquired from patients to staff and from staff and visa-versa as they visit many patients. It can be thus controlled by the better quality of care. Staffing level and advanced nursing education, both variables have strong association to minimize (control) nosocomial infection. Increasing professional knowledge and skills help to follow the medical procedure strictly when helping clients. In case of low staff, nurses have to move elderly next to other elderly and there is more risk of spreading infection, if adequate staff is available then there is low risk of nosocomial infection in custodial setting. Odds ratio of staffing level indicates adequate staff is 1.167 times more likely to reduce this risk and it will happen.

DISCUSSION OF THE FINDINGS

Elder carers and care assistants undergo training in different areas of nursing they have less time or fewer opportunities to upgrade their qualification upon completion of their education or when working to provide better care. Those who have a strong commitment to enhance their knowledge and skills engage in and off-the-job training programs according to their educational level and interest in a specific area of nursing. This is commensurate with an increase in a nurse's advanced training that could encourage health workers to seek further education and professional development in the profession.

In Canada there are many opportunities to further the educational training towards higher educational qualifications, especially those who already have a bachelor's degree. Many nurses with a basic level of education would allow them to move forward and be able to receive additional training towards a master's and doctoral degrees in geriatrics for their career advancement. Thus assessing care for older adults in relation to quality of life is easier among those living in elder homes under long-term care because they have much more controlled environments.

We believe that a sufficient number of trained health workers will provide quality care to older adults. The national data we obtained suggest the qualification and work experience were less likely to have undergone an advanced training, on-site professional development programs without the disruption of the work regimen of healthcare workers and care for older adults would encourage health workers to commit themselves and open the trajectory for career advancement. The increase in care needs and shortage of skilled nursing staff has become a compelling healthcare issue in home care sector in Canada. To address this issue, it may be beneficial to recruit skilled healthcare workers or provide further training to low skilled healthcare workers to meet home care demands.

Older adults have emotional attachment to their homes and spend most of their adult lives in their homes. Any sort of change to the ecosystem will lead to an adverse experience and deterioration of the level of their physical ability and thus can result in a lack of independence. These conditions may also cause the disintegration and restriction of living space activities and, in extreme circumstances, a process of early institutionalization (Perez et al., 2001). To compensate, health workers play a role especially in supporting older adults to adjust to their new living environment (Lu & Chang, 1997). The results of this study clearly indicated that to enhance quality of life, health workers' role is important in improving the lives of older adults in Canada and other developed nations. Therefore, improving their work through either attending trainings within or outside the institution in which they work or completing an advanced education is necessary to understand perform and improve the quality of health system in Canada.

FUTURE OUTLOOK

With the increased percentage of elderly in Canada it has brought greater need of elderly homes. Certainly, there is a need to scale the training and development of elderly care professionals in Canada and globally, particularly in countries with ageing population. However, the increasing pressure on the primary care and continuing care networks has demanded the reorganization and re-education of care. A national health strategy should adopt an aggressive stance to recruit, sustain, and continuously train health workers. The health system shortage of health workers and increase targets for professional development and sustenance. Currently, Canada relies on immigrant health workers. With immigration laws becoming tighter in Canada (Stewart et al., 2006), the need to provide further education and recruitment of health workers in Canada is quite immense. In addition, bringing informal workers into the formal sector through training and retraining is probably bringing informal workers such efforts benefit the economy at large and helps raise funds that is already stressing the Medicare and Extended Care. Medicare is the universal coverage for all citizens or residents of Canada for necessary hospital and physician services and it is provided on the basis of need, not by financial means (Canadian Healthcare Organization, 2007: Ridic Gleason and Ridic, 2012).

Extended Care, which includes long-term care, is provided based on income, and is not universally covered. Long-term care is not covered under the Canada Health Act, therefore, it is not available to Canadians on a universal basis. However, there are a number of government programs aimed at assisting Canadians with long-term care needs. These programs vary from province to province and are typically based on income (Life 2012). The government covers half of the long-term care costs (Torjman, 2013). The federal government transfers funds to the provinces and territories under health and social transfers to support long-term care services. An efficient and effective high quality service could help in cost-cutting initiatives.

All said than done, according Bergman et al., (1997) care for the elderly in Canada is characterized by fragmentation, lack of overall responsibility, accountability, and negative incentives. Given the limited health workers and growing older population in Canada; the diverse agencies, jurisdictions and professionals which include homecare and volunteer agencies, day centers and long-term care centers. Each entity has its own policies, regulation and type of services. Each institution has its own standards to attract, retain and train health workers. This process shall allow for greater accessibility for greater data on elderly carers in Canada. It was shown in this study that quality health significantly improves the quality of life in elderly whether in reducing injury, reducing medical administration errors or even nosocomial infections. Strategic development and future directions need to focus on quality issues and health promotion and geriatrics education and post basic education. The development of the health systems must also adapt to meet the growing needs of old persons for long-term care, when the system is not an abler to accommodate for both long stay in elderly homes, other models of home-based and facility-based places are being used as alternative models of home care. One such initiative is the Quebec's Ministry of Health and Social Services developed a model for a system of integrated care for the frail elderly (Système de services intégrés pour personnes âgées en perte d'antonomie [SIPA]). Such a system is designed around the community-based primary care system based on a patient-focused model designed to assure comprehensive care, integration of all available services and continuity of care for needy elderly. SIPA model allows for a one entry place for care in which the elderly receives medical treatment or palliative care or long-stay boarding (Beland, Bergman, & Lebel, 2000). Such initiatives and others could allow for mainstreaming old people's issues into national development plans. Too often strategies and action plans are aborted or shelved and not implemented because of lack of funding. Putting these isssues in legistlation and national development plans helps raising them high on national agenda and securing the budget needed for sustainable implementation of the plans. Significanitly, these inititatives, should be connected to strengthening the health care system to provide equitable access to health care services for all, including old people, allows to stress on the education and re-education of health workers particularly focusing on health promotion, disease prevention and early screening.

REFERENCES

Aiken, L. H. Cimiotti, J. P., Sloane, D. M., Smith, H. L., Flynn, L., Neff, D. F. (2011). The effects of nurse staffing and nurse education on patient deaths in hospitals with different nurse work environments. *Medical Care*, *49*(12), 104. https://doi.org/10.1097/MLR.0b013e318 2330b6e.

Aiken, L. H., Clarke, S. P., Cheung, R. B., Sloane, D. M., & Silber, J. H. (2003). Educational levels of nurses and surgical patient mortality. *JAMA, 290*(12), 1617-1623. https://doi.org/10.1001/jama.290.12.1617.

Aylward, S., Stolee P., Keat N., Johncox V. (2003). Effectiveness of continuing education in long-term care: a literature review. *The Gerontologist*, *43*(2), 259-271. https://doi.org/10.1093/geront/43.2.259.

Bartels, Y. Anke, S. Denise P. (2012) Higher Education in Nursing-demand and supply-results of an exploratory qualitative analysis in German, *Pflegewissenschaft*, 14(10): 548-58.

Beland, F., Bergman, H., & Lebel, P. (2000). Système de services intégrés pour personnes âgées en perte d'autonomie. Évaluation de la phase I. [Integrated service system for the elderly with loss of autonomy. Phase I evaluation.] *Groupe de recherche, Université McGill et Université de Montréal (GR-SIPA), Montréal.*

Bergman, H., Béland, F., Lebel, P., Contandriopoulos, A. P., Tousignant, P., Brunelle, Y., ... & Clarfield, M. (1997). Care for Canada's frail elderly population: fragmentation or integration?. *CMAJ*, *157*(8):1116-1121.

Beth, N. (Jan 23, 2019). *The Evolution of nursing education - is today's education preparing nurses for tomorrow's growing health challenges?* AllNurses, Magazine, Bloomington, MN: allnurses.com.

Burau, V. D., Theobald, H., & Blank, R. H. (2007). *Governing home care: A cross-national comparison*. Edward Elgar Publishing.

C. D. Howe Institute (2013). *Long-Term Care for the Elderly: Challenges and Policy Option*; Commentary NO. 367.

Canadian Healthcare Organization (2007) *Canadian Health Care: Health Care Funding*, http://www.canadian-healthcare.org/page8.html.

Canadian National *Survey of the Work and Health of Nurses* (NSWHN) (2005). Retrieved in November 22, 2011 from http://www23.statcan.

gc.ca/imdb/p2SV.pl?Function=getSurvey&SDDS=5080&Item_Id=13648.

Canadian Nurses Association (2015) *Becoming an RN: Registered Nurses a leading force for change*: https://www.cna-aiic.ca/en/becoming-an-rn.

Cesari, M., Landi, F., Torre, S., Onder, G., Lattanzio, F., & Bernabei, R. (2002). Prevalence and risk factors for falls in an older community-dwelling population. *The Journals of Gerontology Series A: Biological Sciences and Medical Sciences*, 57(11), M722-M726.

Canadian Institute for Health Information (2010). *Regulated nurses: Canadian trends, 2005 to 2009.* (Nursing Report). Available from: https://secure.cihi.ca/free_products/nursing_report_2005-2009_en.pdf.

Canadian Institute of Health Information (2012) *Health Care in Canada 2012: A focus on wait time.* Available from: https://secure.cihi.ca/free_products/HCIC2012-FullReport-ENweb.pdf.

Department of Health, London, (2007) *Departmental Report: The Health and Personal Social Services Programmes.*

Donabedian, A. (1966) Evaluating the quality of medical care. *The Milbank Memorial Fund Quarterly*, 44:166-206. doi: 10.2307/334 8969.

Estabrooks, C. A., Midodzi, W. K., Cummings, G. C., Ricker, K. L. & Giovanetti, P. (2005) The impact of hospital nursing characteristics on 30-day mortality. *Nursing Research*, 54(2), 72-84.

Feletti, F. and Sanson-Fisher, R. (1986). Patient satisfaction with primary-care consultations *Journal of Behavioral Medicine* August 9, (4):389–399.

Health Force Ontario Canada (2015) *Entry to Practice Requirement for Nurses.* Available from http://www.healthforceontario.ca/en/Home/Nurses/Training_|_Practising_Outside_Ontario/Practice Requirements.

Henderson, V. (2006) The Concept of Nursing: *Journal of Advanced Nursing* 53(1) 21-34.

Johansson, L (2005) *Current Developments in Care of the Elderly in Sweden.* The Swedish National Board of Health and Welfare. http://www.socialstyrelsen.se.

Institute of Medicine (1999) *To Err is Human: Building a Safer Health System*, Washington, DC: National Academies Press USA.

Kane RA, Kane RL, Ladd R. (1998) *The heart of long-term care*. New York: Oxford University Press.

Kong, F. (2018). Aging trend of the world. In *The Structure of Healthy Life Determinants* (pp. 7-21). Springer, Singapore.

Li, S., & Kenward, K. (2006). *A national survey on elements of nursing education* (pp. 1-4). Chicago, IL: National Council of State Boards of Nursing.

Life, C. (2010). Health Insurance Association Inc. 2012. *CLHIA report on long-term care policy: improving the accessibility, quality and sustainability of long-term care in Canada, 4.*

Linda H., Sean P., R., Obyn B., Douglas M and Jeffrey H. (2003) Educational Levels of Hospital Nurses and Surgical Patient Mortality, *JAMA*, 290(12). doi:10.1001/jama.290.12.1617.

Lu, L. & Chang, C. J. (1997). Social Support, Health and Satisfaction among the Elderly with Chronic Conditions in Taiwan. *Journal of Health Psychology, 2*(4), 471-80. https://doi.org/10.1177/135910539700200404.

Mays & Pope, 2000) *Qualitative research in health care* BMJ *2000;* 320: 50. doi: https://doi.org/10.1136/bmj.320.7226.50.

McDonald, K. M., Sundaram, V., Bravata, D. M., Lewis, R., Lin, N., Kraft, S. A., ... & Owens, D. K. (2007). *Closing the quality gap: a critical analysis of quality improvement strategies* (Vol. 7: Care Coordination).

Merriam Webster Dictionary (2020) *Definition Of Health Care*: Retrieved From Https://Www.Merriam-Webster.Com/Dictionary/Health%20care.

OECD (2014) *OECD Health Statistics* 2014 http://www.oecd.org/els/health-systems/health-data.htm.

Perez, F., Fernandez, G., Rivera, E. & Rojo Abuin, J. (2001). Ageing in Place: Predictors of the Residential Satisfaction of Elderly. *Social Indicators Research, 54*(2), 173–208. https://doi.org/10.1023/A:1010852607362.

Ridic, G., Gleason, S. and Ridic, O. (2012) Comparisons of Health Care Systems in the United States, Germany and Canada, *Materia Socio Medica*, 2012 Jun; 24(2): 112-120.

Rosseter, R (2012) *Creating a More Highly Qualified Nursing Workforce, Doctootral Dissertation*, Walden University Retrieved from: http://www.aacn.nche.edu/media-relations/fact-sheets/nursing-workforce.

Statistics Canada (2014) *Population and Family Estimation Methods at Statistics Canada.* Minister of Industry.

Statistics Canada (2016) *Population and Family Estimation Methods at Statistics Canada.* Minister of Industry.

Stewart, I., Barnes-Holmes, D., Barnes-Holmes, Y., Bond, F. W., & Hayes, S. C. (2006). Relational Frame Theory and Industrial/Organizational Psychology. In S. C. Hayes, F. W. Bond, D. Barnes-Holmes, & J. Austin (Eds.), *Acceptance and Mindfulness at Work: Applying Acceptance and Commitment Therapy and Relational Frame Theory to Organizational Behavior Management* (pp. 55-90). Binghamton, NY: The Haworth.

Tourangeau, A. E., Doran, D. M., Hall, L. M., O'Brien Pallas, L., Pringle, D., Tu, J. V., & Cranley, L. A. (2007). Impact of hospital nursing care on 30-day mortality for acute medical patients. *Journal of advanced nursing*, *57*(1), 32-44. https://doi.org/10.1111/j.1365-2648.2006.04084.x.

Torjman, S. (2013) *Financing Long-Term Care: More Money in the Mix,* Ottawa, ON: The Caledon Institute of Social Policy.

Urquhart, A., Kimpton, C. P., Downes, T. J., & Gill, P. (1994). Variation in short tandem repeat sequences—a survey of twelve microsatellite loci for use as forensic identification markers. *International journal of legal medicine*, *107*(1), 13-20. https://doi.org/10.1007/BF01247268.

United Nations. Department of International Economic, United Nations. Department for Economic, Social Information, & Policy Analysis. (1999). *World population prospects* (Vol. 2). United Nations, Department of International, Economic and Social Affairs.

World Health Organization (2006) Strategies for assisting health workers to modify and improve skills: Developing quality health care - a process of change. *Issues in health services delivery Discussion paper No. 1.*

Williams, A. P., Peckham, A., Kuluski, K., Montgomery, R., Morton, F., & Watkins, J. (2010). *Formal and informal care for older persons:*

Assessing the balance in Ontario. Canadian Research Network for Care in the Community.

In: Elderly Care
Editor: Sean M. Eckstein ISBN: 978-1-53618-446-4

Chapter 6

INTERNATIONAL PERSPECTIVES REGARDING FUTURE DEVELOPMENT IN NURSING HOMES: HONG KONG, JAPAN, AND GERMANY

Shuk Kwan Tang*[1]*, Mimi M. Y. Tse*[1]*,
***Noriko Yamamoto-Mitani*[2] *and Andrea Budnick*[3]**
[1]School of Nursing, The Hong Kong Polytechnic University, Hong Kong SAR
[2]School of Nursing, University of Tokyo, Tokyo, Japan
[3]Charité, Universitätsmedizin Berlin, Institute of Medical Sociology and Rehabilitation Science, Berlin, Germany

ABSTRACT

The services and care delivered to older adults is often a concern of the community and policy makers. Populations worldwide are aging rapidly and life expectancies are growing. The demand for elderly services to provide support and care to older adults in the community is growing, as is the demand for nursing homes. Governments and societies have to plan for adequate facilities and manpower to provide quality care to their populations. The opinions of the aging population regarding nursing homes should also be taken into consideration. For future planning, the perspectives of middle-aged adults should also be included. They are the older adults and service users of the future. In this chapter, an overview of the aging populations in Hong Kong, Japan, and Germany are presented. The perceptions of nursing homes held by older and middle-aged adults, and their expectations of what nursing homes will be like in the future are explored.

INTRODUCTION

Aging is a process that cannot be prevented. Deterioration in physical and psychological health is a common problem of aging. Older adults may be no longer be able to age in place and may need to move into a nursing home to receive care from healthcare professionals. As the aging population is increasing in proportion to the total population, the demand for nursing homes is growing. However, the wishes of older adults may be neglected. Whether they are willing to stay in a nursing home and what their expectations of nursing homes are, need to be addressed.

Around the world, populations are aging rapidly. It is estimated that by 2050, one out of six people in the world will be over the age of 65 (16%) (United Nations, 2019). At that time, the size of the aged population will be double that of 2015, at 2.1 billion (United Nations, 2015). Aging is a global challenge. Life expectancies have been increasing since World War II, and now exceed 74 years in East Asia (National Institute on Aging, Naitonal Institute of Health, & World Health Organization, 2011).

Hong Kong's Aging Population

The aging population in Hong Kong has similar characteristics to those of other countries. The term "older adults" usually refers to people aged 65 or above, and this is the definition that the Hong Kong government uses to plan its services for the elderly (Census and Statistics Department, 2018). The aging population is growing at a rapid pace. The total number of older adults in 2016 was 1,163,153, an increase of 36.4% compared to 2006. The percentage increase in the number of older adults aged 80 or above was 66.7% over the last decade (Census and Statistics Department, 2018).

According to the 2016 Population By-census, 91.9% of older adults lived in their own home and 8.1% lived in non-domestic households. Non-domestic households include homes for the aged, hospitals, penal institutions, and other types of institutions. There was a trebling in the number of foreign domestic helpers hired in households with older adults. The number of households made up of only older adults increased by 67.4%. A high percentage of internal migration involved older adults (37.1%), which can be related to their move from a household to a nursing home (Census and Statistics Department, 2018). The proportion of households hiring helpers, the proportion with older adults, and the number of older adults moving to nursing homes will continue to grow as the population ages.

Japan's Aging Population

The percentage of individuals aged 65 or over is currently 28.1% in Japan (Statistics Bureau, 2018), the highest in the world (Global Note, 2019). One characteristic of the aging population in Japan is that 14.2% of the population is over the age of 75, which is higher than in any other country (Cabinet House, 2019). The increase in the older-old population means that it is necessary to develop a cost-effective elderly support system.

Germany's Aging Population

Demographic change in Germany is continuing to occur with the increase in life expectancies. Currently, those 65 years of age and older make up 18% of the population; the percentage is expected to grow to 23% by 2060. This will eventually lead to an increase in the number of care-dependent people, because the risk of care dependency increases continuously after the age of 65 (Federal Statistical Office, 2018a).

In Germany, 3.4 million people are officially registered as care dependent. Of this number, 76% are predominantly being cared for at home by a family caregiver, while 24% are receiving care in a nursing home (Federal Statistical Office, 2018b).

Nursing Home Situations

To face the service and care needs of an aging population, adequate residential care facilities have to be developed and run. The Social Welfare Department of the Hong Kong SAR government supervises a residential care service. This service includes homes for the aged, care and attention homes for the elderly, and nursing homes. The admission criteria for the scheme are older adults aged 65 or above who cannot be cared for at home for personal, social, health, and/or other reasons (Social Welfare Department, 2018). The service is provided in the public and private sectors. The number of applications for a place in one of these government-subsidized homes has reached 42,763 as at 31 August 2019. The overall waiting time is 21 months (Social Welfare Department, 2019b). However, only a total of 32,677 places are available (Social Welfare Department, 2019a). It is critical to manage the demand for and supply of this residential service.

In Japan, various residential care services are available under either long-term care insurance (LTCI) or medical care insurance. The fees paid for using welfare facilities for the elderly, healthcare facilities for the elderly, sanatorium-type medical care facilities, and group homes for persons with dementia are reimbursed by LTCI. Some medical facilities include long-term care beds, the fees for which are reimbursed under medical care insurance. These various facilities are used according to the condition of the individual elderly person, and will depend on how much help an individual needs with the activities of daily living, on their level of dementia, or on their need for skilled nursing care. In 2017, there were 7,891 welfare facilities for the elderly (542,498 beds), 4,322 healthcare facilities for the elderly (372,679 beds), 1,196 sanatorium-type medical care facilities (53,352 beds), and 13,346 group homes for persons with dementia (Social Statistics Office, 2018). In 2018, there were 4,583 medical facilities with a total of 328,015 long-term care beds (Health Statistics Office, 2019).

Since the introduction of Volume XI of the German Social Security Code (long-term care insurance) in 1995, the number of care-dependent people has increased steadily. This development is in line with the changes that have been taking place in society, e.g., a decrease in the number of adult children who can take on the role of domestic caregiver (Bundesinstitut für Bevölkerungsforschung, 2019). Moreover, there is a decrease in the willingness of older people to live in conventional nursing homes, and a strong belief in the necessity for self-determination, privacy, and individuality, but also a lack of qualified staff in nursing homes. This raises the question of how to ensure nursing home care for individuals in the future? On the one hand, the results of the study show that older adults in need of care prefer to live independently for as long as possible (Kuhlmey, Dräger, Winter, & Beikirch, 2010). On the other hand, there are in a historical perspective increased requirements of older adults regarding a life in a nursing home (Höpflinger, 2012).

WHAT PERCEPTIONS DO OLDER ADULTS HAVE OF NURSING HOMES?

Older adults viewed entering a nursing home as posing "at least some threat to their self-autonomy and to life itself" (Baldwin, Dendle, & McKinlay, 2019). They enjoyed having control over their daily activities. It gave them a sense of autonomy. Living at home helped them to sustain a self-identity. Home was a place that was full of their memories, whether good or bad. They were able to present themselves as independent, which was meaningful to them (Stones & Gullifer, 2016). When older adults moved into a nursing home, they were away from home and thought they had lost what they had. The experiences of residents in nursing homes may explain why older adults said that they preferred to age in place. They felt a sense of "loss and suffering" and passively accepted their life in a nursing home (Lee, Woo, & Mackenzie, 2002).

Another reason for older adults to resist living in a nursing home may be related to their expectations of the quality of life in these homes. Their quality of life was affected by their level of independence, individuality, and autonomy. An ability to communicate with others, provide self-care, and help others were the factors contributing to a good quality of life. Older adults preferred to have a private room, environmental safety, and security (Lee, Yu, & Kwong, 2009). However, not all nursing home residents are able to stay in a private room. Where rooms are shared, older adults are concerned about the issue of privacy.

THE FUTURE OF CARE FOR AN AGING POPULATION

In Western countries, senior co-housing arrangements are emerging. The concept matches the preference of older adults to age in place (Baldwin et al., 2019). Co-housing refers to the attempt to "mix private and shared living spaces in a way that meets the need for both privacy and a sense of community and support" (Riedy, McKenna, Wynne, & Daly, 2017). It is "an approach to living that is focused on community" (Institute for Sustainable Futures, 2019). Residents design the co-housing arrangement. They are self-governing and actively participate in the community. They share facilities. Co-housing allows for social contacts and encourages community interaction. There are advantages to letting older adults stay in co-housing arrangements, for example, in terms of the provision of informal care, the centralization of resources, the ability to age in place, and the increase in social contacts among the older adults (Institute for Sustainable Futures, 2017).

Ten middle-aged adults (seven females and three males) ranging in age from 45 to 65 were asked about their views and preference for aging in place or living in a nursing home when they become old. Most said that they would like to stay at home when they get old. Only one participant would choose to live in a nursing home. They aimed for independence in choosing to stay at home. They perceived themselves as having good social relationships and a good economic status. They had good appetites and thought that they could maintain good health when they became old. To meet the high demand for aging at home, the Hong Kong Housing Society has a Senior Citizen Residences Scheme to promote "healthy aging" and "aging in place" (Hong Kong Housing Society, 2017c). The scheme involves two buildings in two districts. Each building has self-contained flats with different facilities to fit different levels of dependency and frailty. The emphasis is on "safety, security, identity and comfort" (Hong Kong Housing Society, 2017b). Leisure and cultural facilities, as well medical and health facilities are available (Hong Kong Housing Society, 2017a). At the moment, all units are occupied. A privately owned building with a similar concept is being developed (Ventria Residence, 2019). The demand for such a service has been noticed. The non-institutional design and concepts match the expectations of the currently middle-aged regarding their future needs when they become part of the aged population.

The participants welcomed this idea of co-housing. They were willing to move into a co-housing arrangement when they become old. Co-housing has been developing in Germany, the United Kingdom, the United States, and Australia since the 1970s, starting on a small scale (Ache & Fedrowitz, 2012; Jarvis, 2015). Co-housing arrangements are now found in other countries and continue to expand (Labit, 2015).

To further meet the challenge of caring for increasing numbers of older adults in need of care, in 2015 the Japanese government began promoting a "community-based integrated care system" (Song & Tang, 2019). This is a comprehensive system involving multiple services/facilities located in the community, including hospitals, nursing homes, and residential care facilities. In the promotion of the community-based integrated care system, even those facilities that used to provide traditional long-term, residential care services are now being given financial incentives to send elderly residents back home if they are able to return. Apart from traditional residential care facilities, there are also multiple arrangements/programs that help elderly persons to stay at home for as long as possible, such as small-scale multi-functional services in the community, where some temporary residential care services are available. In 2017, there were 5,342 small-scale multi-functional services (Social Statistics Office, 2018). Thus, residential care homes and nursing homes are now operationalized within the integrated care system in close connection with the community.

With regard to nursing home care in Germany in the future, it is conceivable that central units (e.g., a large kitchen) may no longer exist, but older adults residing in nursing homes might live independently in single apartments while a complex offering structured activities exists, which can be taken advantage of if necessary. Furthermore, new technologies, useful for both nursing home staff and residents, should be integrated in daily nursing care. On this, there is a great need for research (Zwick et al. 2019).

CONCLUSION

The aged population of the future prefers co-housing. This concept fits with the needs of a generation that aims to have areas for both privacy and social contact. Their opinions should be taken into account by policy makers. They will be of help to society in planning for long-term healthcare services for an aging population. The idea of co-housing is growing in popularity worldwide, including in Hong Kong, Japan, and Germany. The successful examples and experiences of developing co-housing in other countries should be shared. The benefits of co-housing should be emphasized and promoted. The concept of co-housing and the possibility of implementing it in the community should be further explored in Hong Kong.

REFERENCES

Ache, P., & Fedrowitz, M. (2012). The development of co-housing initiatives in Germany. *Built Environment, 38*(3), 395-412.

Baldwin, C., Dendle, K., & McKinlay, A. (2019). Initiating senior co-housing: people, place, and long-term security. *Journal of Housing For the Elderly*, 1-24. doi: 10.1080/02763893.2019.1583152.

Bundesinstitut für Bevölkerungsforschung. (2019). *Zusammengefasste Geburtenziffer in Deutschland, 1871 bis 2016* [*Total birth rate in Germany, 1871 to 2016*]. Retrieved from https://www.bib.bund.de/DE/Fakten/Fakt/F08-Zusammengefasste-Geburtenziffer-ab-1871.html.

Cabinet House. (2019). *Reiwa Gannen Kourei Syakai Hakusho (White paper on aging society in 2019) (in Japanese).* Author.

Census and Statistics Department. (2018). *2016 Population By-census - Thematic report: Older persons*. Retrieved from Hong Kong SAR: https://www.bycensus2016.gov.hk/data/16BC_Older_persons_report.pdf.

Federal Statistical Office (2018a). *Pflegestatistik 2017 – Statistical analysis about nursing and care.* Wiesbaden: Statistisches Bundesamt, 2018: p.20.

Federal Statistical Office (2018b). *Pflegestatistik 2017 – Statistical analysis about nursing and care.* Wiesbaden: Statistisches Bundesamt, 2018: p.16.

Global Note. (2019). *Sekai no Koureika ritsu: Kokusai Hikaku (Aging of the world: international comparison) (in Japanese).* Downloaded from https://www.globalnote.jp/ on 10/12/2019.

Health Statistics Office. (2019). *Hospital Report.* Author.

Höpflinger, F. (2012). Household and living in old age – its historical changes. *Age Dossier*, 4-11.

Hong Kong Housing Society. (2017a, 2017). *Background - Benefits to customers*. Retrieved from https://www.hkhs.com/sen_20040903/eng/cheerful_court/background/bentocus.htm

Hong Kong Housing Society. (2017b, 2017). *Background - Design.* Retrieved from https://www.hkhs.com/sen_20040903/eng/cheerful_court/background/design.htm.

Hong Kong Housing Society. (2017c, 2017). *Background - Executive summary.* Retrieved from https://www.hkhs.com/sen_20040903/eng/cheerful_court/background/exesum.htm.

Institute for Sustainable Futures. (2017). *Cohousing for seniors: Literature review.* Retrieved from https://www.uts.edu.au/sites/default/files/article/downloads/Cohousing%20for%20Seniors_Lit%20Review.pdf.

Institute for Sustainable Futures. (2019). *Cohousing for seniors: What is cohousing?* Retrieved from https://www.uts.edu.au/sites/default/files/article/downloads/UTS_ISF_What_Is_Cohousing_factsheet_WEB.pdf

Jarvis, H. (2015). Towards a deeper understanding of the social architecture of co-housing: evidence from the UK, USA and Australia. *Urban Research & Practice, 8*(1), 93-105.

Kuhlmey, A., Dräger, D., Winter, M., & Beikirch, E. (2010). COMPASS – Questioning regarding expectations and wishes of a qualitative good care. *Informationsdienst altersfragen, 37*(4), 4-11.

Labit, A. (2015). Self-managed co-housing in the context of an ageing population in Europe. *Urban Research & Practice, 8*(1), 32-45.

Lee, D. T., Woo, J., & Mackenzie, A. E. (2002). A review of older people's experiences with residential care placement. *Journal of Advanced Nursing, 37*(1), 19-27.

Lee, D. T., Yu, D. S., & Kwong, A. N. (2009). Quality of life of older people in residential care home: A literature review. *Journal of Nursing and Healthcare of Chronic Illness, 1*(2), 116-125. doi: 10.1111/j.1752-9824.2009.01018.x.

National Institute on Aging, Naitonal Institute of Health, & World Health Organization. (2011). *Global health and aging*. Retrieved from https://www.nia.nih.gov/sites/default/files/2017-06/global_health_aging.pdf.

Riedy, C., McKenna, K., Wynne, L., & Daly, M. (2017). *Co-housing works well for older people, once they get past the image problem*. Retrieved from https://theconversation.com/co-housing-works-well-for-older-people-once-they-get-past-the-image-problem-79907.

Social Statistics Office. (2018). *Survey of Institutions and Establishments for Long-term Care.* Author.

Social Welfare Department. (2018). Residential care services for elders. In *Hong Kong SAR* (Ed.). Hong Kong SAR: Social Welfare Department.

Social Welfare Department. (2019a, September 11 2019). *Overview of residential care services for the elderly.* Retrieved from https://www.swd.gov.hk/en/index/site_pubsvc/page_elderly/sub_residentia/id_overviewon/

Social Welfare Department. (2019b, August 31 2019). *Statistics on 'Waiting list for subsidised residential care services for the elderly', 'Waiting time for residential care services' and 'Turn for placement offer for cases applying for residential care services'* Retrieved from https://www.swd.gov.hk/storage/asset/section/632/en/LTC_statistics_HP-Eng(201908).pdf.

Song P, Tang W. (2019). The community-based integrated care system in Japan: Health care and nursing care challenges posed by super-aged society. *Biosci Trends.* 13(3):279-281. doi: 10.5582/bst.2019.01173.

Statistics Bureau of Japan. (2018). Population Census. Author.

Stones, D., & Gullifer, J. (2016). 'At home it's just so much easier to be yourself': Older adults' perceptions of ageing in place. *Ageing & Society, 36*(3), 449-481.

United Nations. (2015). *World population ageing.* Retrieved from New York: https://www.un.org/en/development/desa/population/publications/pdf/ageing/WPA2015_Report.pdf.

United Nations. (2019). *Ageing.* Retrieved from https://www.un.org/en/sections/issues-depth/ageing/

Ventria Residence. (2019, 2019). *Mission - Ventria Residence.* Retrieved from https://www.ventriaresidence.com/en/mission/

Zwick, M.M., Hampel, J. (2019) Cui bono? A debate on the pros and cons of robotics in nursing care. *Zeitschrift für Technikfolgenabschätzung in Theorie und Praxis*, 28(2): 52-57.

In: Elderly Care
Editor: Sean M. Eckstein
ISBN: 978-1-53618-446-4

Chapter 7

OLDER ADULTS LIVING IN NURSING HOMES: CAN WE DO SOMETHING TO ENHANCE THEIR HAPPINESS AND REDUCE THEIR PAIN?

Mimi Tse[1,*], Shamay NG[2], Xue Bai[3], Paul Lee[4], Raymond Lo[5] and Shuk Kwan Tang[6]

[1]Associate Professor, School of Nursing, The Hong Kong Polytechnic University, Hong Kong SAR

[2]2Professor, Department of Rehabilitation Sciences, The Hong Kong Polytechnic University, Hong Kong SAR

[3]3Associate Professor, Department of Applied Social Sciences, The Hong Kong Polytechnic University, Hong Kong SAR

[4]4Assistant Professor, School of Nursing, The Hong Kong Polytechnic University, Hong Kong SAR

[5]Consultant Physician, Department of Geriatrics and Palliative Medicine, Shatin Hospital, Hospital Authority, Hong Kong SAR

[6]Clinical Instructor, School of Nursing, The Hong Kong Polytechnic University, Hong Kong SAR

[*] Corresponding Author's Email: mimi.tse@polyu.edu.hk; Tel.: +852 2766 6541.

Abstract

Pain is common in older adults, and can lead to various physical and psychological issues. Pain and pain-related situations among elderly people living in nursing homes are even more serious. In this chapter, we report the effects of pain situations and a non-drug pain management program for older adults in a nursing home environment.

Background

Because of the physiological changes associated with aging, older people are more susceptible to various kinds of diseases (Brochet, Michel, Barberger-Gateau, & DARTIGUES, 1998; Rosenthal & Kavic, 2004; Thomas, Peat, Harris, Wilkie, & Croft, 2004). Indeed, most age-related diseases and illnesses bring chronic pain and disability.

Chronic non-cancer pain is common among older adults and is often associated with significant physical and psychosocial incapacities (Brochet, Michel, Barberger-Gateau, & DARTIGUES, 1998; Rosenthal & Kavic, 2004; Thomas, Peat, Harris, Wilkie, & Croft, 2004). Older adults with pain are more depressed, anxious, and have reduced social interaction (Brochet et al., 1998; Rosenthal & Kavic, 2004; Thomas et al., 2004). Pain in older adults tends to be constant in nature, moderate to severe in intensity, and years long in duration (Brochet et al., 1998; Chung & Wong, 2007). The prevalence of pain among nursing home residents is as high as 70%-80% (Brochet et al., 1998; Thomas et al., 2004). Chronic pain is regarded as pain that persists past the normal time of healing (Bonica & Hoffman, 1954). Three months is the most convenient point of division between acute and chronic pain for nonmalignant pain (Merskey & Bogduk, 1994).

Chronic pain is common in later life and is associated with negative mood states and life satisfaction (Closs, 2007). Many older people accept pain as part of their life and do not seek help until it becomes severe and unbearable (Closs, 2007; Ferrell, 1991). The consequences of chronic pain among older people are considerable and include loneliness, social isolation, depression, impaired functional mobility and ambulation, and increased healthcare utilization and costs (Yonan & Wegener, 2003). Older people with chronic pain tend to become isolated and unwilling to go out and meet friends and family members; they are also less likely to express their feelings and thus more likely to become lonely. This may create misunderstandings and even interpersonal conflicts among family members and friends who are caring for them (Cann, 2008).

These negative impacts of chronic pain are more disturbing for older people in residential care. Nursing home residents are physically frail, live in "closed" nursing home environments, and may have difficulty seeking pain management strategies. Moreover, Chinese older adults are often unwilling to report their pain to healthcare professionals,5 making the need to provide pain management education to nursing home residents a high priority.

Pain is often inadequately managed (Chung & Wong, 2007). Analgesics remain the primary approach to managing pain (Tse, Pun, & Benzie, 2005). Yet older adults worry about adverse reactions to drugs and accept chronic pain as part of aging (Brochet et al., 1998; Chung & Wong, 2007; Thomas et al., 2004). Non-pharmacological strategies, including pain education programs, exercise programs, massage, relaxation therapies, cognitive-behavioural therapy, listening to music, visual stimulation, and motivational interviewing, are becoming increasingly popular (Rosenthal & Kavic, 2004).

Self-management is essential for optimal outcomes in chronic disease management. Self-management is "the ability to manage the symptoms, treatment, physical and psychosocial consequences and lifestyle changes inherent in living with a chronic condition (Bonica, 1953)." Pain self-management interventions using nonpharmacological strategies have been shown to be effective among older adults (Bonica & Hoffman, 1954; Merskey & Bogduk, 1994), yet there is still no clear consensus regarding the best nonpharmacological pain treatment for this population (Bonica & Hoffman, 1954; Merskey & Bogduk, 1994; Tse et al., 2005).

With funding from the Jockey Club, the research team adopted Ersek's (Closs, 2007) chronic pain self-management program on nursing homes residents (Ferrell, 1991). Significant reductions in pain and improvements in physical and psychological parameters were found as compared to the control group (Ferrell, 1991). In this chapter, we discuss details of this non-drug pain management programme.

INTERVENTION: NON-DRUG PAIN MANAGEMENT PROGRAMME

The Stanford Chronic Disease Self-Management Program and the chronic pain self-management program developed by Ersek et al. (Closs, 2007) were used as our theoretical framework, with a focus on the ability to manage pain and pain-related symptoms, treatment, physical and psychosocial consequences, and lifestyle changes inherent in living with a chronic pain condition (Bonica & Hoffman, 1954; Closs, 2007; Merskey & Bogduk, 1994). Teaching methods include dialectic lecturing (group), small group discussions, case sharing, and demonstrations and return-demonstrations (individual) on non-pharmacological practices. The instructional model is group-based.

A pain management program (PAP) using a teaching manual (outlined in Appendix 1) was designed. The content was validated by the research team, a geriatric physician consultant specializing in pain, a registered physiotherapist, and an advanced practice nurse experienced in elderly care.

Nursing home residents will undergo one 1-hour session per week for 12 weeks. The PAP will start with 20 minutes of physical exercises performed under the supervision of peer volunteers. This will be followed by 30 minutes of pain management education, including information on pain situations, the impacts of pain, the use of drugs and non-drug strategies for pain management, and demonstrations and return-demonstrations of various non-drug pain management techniques.

APPENDIX 1. PAIN MANAGEMENT PROGRAM (PAP) OUTLINE

Content		Pain Management Program (PAP)	
Week	Physical Exercise (20 minutes)	Interactive teaching and sharing of pain management education (30 minutes)	Portfolio Entry (10 minutes)
1	Correct body posture and alignment, Stretching of arms, legs, and body muscles; Balancing exercise; Shoulder & neck exercise; Hip exercise; Knee exercise; Towel dancing	Pain situations among themselves; Effects of pain in their daily life; Can we do something?	Peer volunteers worked with the participants to make entries on the activity of the day in the "I can do it" booklet.
2		The use of an oral drug: effects & side-effects; labels of oral drugs	
3		The use of a non-drug therapy: Hot pad & cold pad; how to use & safety issues	
4, 5		The use of a non-drug therapy: listening to music	
6, 7		The use of a non-drug therapy: Massage	
8, 9		The use of a non-drug therapy: visual stimulation - watching the natural environment & making a photo album	
10, 11		The use of a non-drug therapy: sense of smell & taste - making a bag of dried flowers & tasting tea	
12		Revision & Wrapping Up	

At the end of the session, the peer volunteers will help the participants make portfolio entries on the activities of the day, to help them recall the various pain relief methods learned in each class (Kwekkeboom, 1999).

Discussion

The management of chronic pain is generally inadequate. Physicians are often reluctant to prescribe adequate analgesic treatments for fear of inducing drug addiction (Corran, Helme, & Gibson, 2001). It was found that over 50% of analgesic medications were ordered on an "as needed" basis (Won et al., 2004). This places the responsibility for pain relief on the sufferer, in that he or she must request it.

Furthermore, the treatment request is likely to be made only when the pain has reached the patient's limit of tolerance. This limits the success of this strategy, because older people generally accept pain as part of growing old, and often fail to ask for pain relief despite experiencing severe pain (Closs, 2007; Prohaska, Keller, Leventhal, & Leventhal, 1987). In this regard, the use of nonprescription, preferably nonpharmacological, pain relief measures is appealing, to reduce the disability and distress associated with chronic pain.

The gate control theory (Melzack & Wall, 1965) describes three dimensions of pain: sensory-discriminative, motivational-affective, and cognitive control. The transmission of nerve impulses to spinal cord transmission cells is modulated by a spinal gating mechanism in the dorsal horn. The spinal gating mechanism is influenced by the amount of activity in large diameter and small-diameter fibers carrying nerve impulses. Activity in the large fibers tends to inhibit transmission, whereas small-fiber activity tends to facilitate transmission. Likewise, the spinal gating mechanism is influenced by nerve impulses that descend from the brain. According to Melzack, selective cognitive processes are activated by a specialized system of large-diameter fibers and have the property of modulating the spinal gating mechanism by the descending fibers. Experimental and clinical studies support the concept of the transmission of pain as being modulated by afferent input from the periphery, descending inhibitory systems, and psychological factors.

It is noted that people aged 80 and over will continue to postpone disabling health problems as long as they maintain a relatively vigorous level of intellectual, interpersonal, and physical activity (Lassey & Lassey, 2001).

In light of the high prevalence of chronic pain and its impact on physical and psychological perspectives among older people, and the inadequate management of chronic pain situations among older persons in residential care, the use of the non-drug pain management program for older adults is highly appealing.

REFERENCES

Bonica, J. J., & Hoffman, J. F. (1954). The Management of Pain with Special Emphasis on the Use of Analgesic Blocks in Diagnosis, Prognosis, and Therapy. *Anesthesia & Analgesia*, 34(5), 57-58.

Brochet, B., Michel, P., Barberger-Gateau, P., & DARTIGUES, J.-F. (1998). Population-based study of pain in elderly people: a descriptive survey. *Age and Ageing*, 27(3), 279-284.

Cann, P. (2008). Pain in older adults should not be seen as part of ageing. *British journal of community nursing*, 13(12), 574-576.

Chung, J. W., & Wong, T. K. (2007). Prevalence of pain in a community population. *Pain Medicine*, 8(3), 235-242.

Closs, S. J. (2007). Assessment of pain, mood and quality of life. *Pain in older people*, 11-19.

Corran, T. M., Helme, R. D., & Gibson, S. J. (2001). Multidisciplinary assessment and treatment of pain in older persons. *Topics in Geriatric Rehabilitation*, 16(3), 1-11.

Ferrell, B. A. (1991). Pain management in elderly people. *Journal of the American Geriatrics Society*, 39(1), 64-73.

Kwekkeboom, K. L. (1999). A model for cognitive-behavioral interventions in cancer pain management. Image: *the Journal of Nursing Scholarship*, 31(2), 151-155.

Lassey, W. R., & Lassey, M. L. (2001). *Quality of life for older people: An international perspective:* Prentice-Hall Incorporated.

Melzack, R., & Wall, P. D. (1965). Pain mechanisms: a new theory. *Science*, 150(3699), 971-979.

Merskey, H., & Bogduk, N. (1994). International Association for the Study of Pain. Task Force on Taxonomy. *Classification of chronic pain: descriptions of chronic pain syndromes and definitions of pain terms*. Seattle; IASP Press.

Prohaska, T. R., Keller, M. L., Leventhal, E. A., & Leventhal, H. (1987). Impact of symptoms and aging attribution on emotions and coping. *Health Psychology*, 6(6), 495.

Rosenthal, R. A., & Kavic, S. M. (2004). Assessment and management of the geriatric patient. *Critical Care Medicine*, 32(4), S92-S105.

Thomas, E., Peat, G., Harris, L., Wilkie, R., & Croft, P. R. (2004). The prevalence of pain and pain interference in a general population of older adults: cross-sectional findings from the North Staffordshire Osteoarthritis Project (NorStOP). *Pain*, 110(1-2), 361-368.

Tse, M. M., Pun, S. P., & Benzie, I. F. (2005). Pain relief strategies used by older people with chronic pain: an exploratory survey for planning patient-centred intervention. *Journal of Clinical Nursing,* 14(3), 315-320.

Won, A. B., Lapane, K. L., Vallow, S., Schein, J., Morris, J. N., & Lipsitz, L. A. (2004). Persistent Nonmalignant Pain and Analgesic Prescribing Patterns in Elderly Nursing Home Residents: (See editorial comments by Dr. Debra Weiner on pp 1020–1022). *Journal of the American Geriatrics Society*, 52(6), 867-874.

Yonan, C. A., & Wegener, S. T. (2003). Assessment and management of pain in the older adult. *Rehabilitation Psychology*, 48(1), 4.

In: Elderly Care
Editor: Sean M. Eckstein
ISBN: 978-1-53618-446-4

Chapter 8

DESPERATE SOULS: MEDICARE HOME CARE IGNORES PATIENT SUBSTANCE ABUSE ASSESSMENT AND TREATMENT

William Cabin[*]
Social Work Department, Temple University, Philadelphia, PA, US

ABSTRACT

There is extensive literature on the significance of substance use, misuse, and abuse among the elderly in the United States. A literature review indicates no studies on the nature, significance, or impacts of the lack of substance use and abuse coverage in Medicare home health. This chapter presents background on the topic and an initial, exploratory study to address the literature gap, based on interviews of a convenience sample of 26 home care social workers between January 2013 and May 2014 in the New York City metropolitan area. Results indicate social workers believe substance use and abuse occurs frequently among Medicare home health patients; substance use and abuse is not assessed and treated professionally in Medicare home health; the lack of coverage in Medicare home health results in exacerbation of existing patient physical and mental

[*] Corresponding Author's Email: wcabin@umich.edu.

health conditions, which, in turn, worsen substance use and abuse conditions; the homebound requirement and lack of coverage of transportation and personal care assistants limits home care patients ability to obtain outpatient substance use and abuse treatment; and lack of home-based assessment and treatment contributes to increased home care readmissions, re-hospitalizations, and increased caregiver burden.

Keywords: medicare, nurses, home health, substance use, substance abuse

INTRODUCTION

Substance use, misuse, and abuse has been documented as a major national problem, accentuated recently by what is commonly referred to as the opioid epidemic (United States Department of Health and Human Services, Office of the Surgeon General 2016, 2018). The Substance Abuse and Mental Health Services Administration (SAMHSA) has reported in 2013 that 9.4% (or 24.6 million) of Americans aged 12 or older had used an illicit drug in the past month, an increase over 8.3% in 2002 (National Institute on Drug Abuse 2019).

According to the United States Department of Health & Human Services (USDHHS 2016), over 175 million persons aged 12 and older (65.7%) reported alcohol use in the past year; more than 36 million (13.5%) reported using marijuana in the past year; 12.5 million reported misusing prescription pain relievers; and over 300,000 reported using heroin in the past year. Almost 8 percent of the population met diagnostic criteria for a substance use disorder (SUD) for alcohol or illicit drugs, and 1 percent met diagnostic criteria for both an alcohol and illicit drug use disorder. USDHHS (2016) further reports that while 20.8 million people (7.8 percent of the population) met the diagnostic criteria for a substance use disorder in 2015, only 2.2 million individuals (10.4 percent) received any type of treatment and only 63.7 percent of those treated received treatment in specialty substance use disorder program.

USDHHS (2018, 5) defines substance misuse as, "The use of any substance in a manner, situation, amount, or frequency that can cause harm to users or to those around them." USDHHS (2018, 5) indicates substance use disorder "Occurs when the recurrent use of alcohol and/or drugs causes clinically and functionally significant impairment, such as health problems, disability, and failure to meet major responsibilities at work, school, or home. According to the Diagnostic and Statistical Manual of Mental Disorder s (DSM)-5, a diagnosis of substance use disorder is based on evidence of impaired control, social impairment, risky use, and pharmacological criteria." However, while Individuals with substance use disorders have elevated rates of substance misuse, such as related health and social problems and costs, many people who misuse substances do not meet the diagnostic criteria for a substance use disorder (USDHHS 2016).

Alcohol misuse, illicit drug use, misuse of medications, and substance use disorders have significant adverse consequences for individuals and society. In the United States alone they result in an estimated $400 billion in lost in workplace productivity (USDHHS 2016). Worldwide, the global burden of disability attributable to substance misuse problems and disorders, mainly due to lost ability to work and years of life lost to premature mortality, is significant. A 2010 international study (Whiteford et al. 2013) found that mental and substance use disorders were the leading causes of years lived with disability worldwide, largely because these problems begin for many individuals early in their lives and can continue, particularly if untreated, for long periods into old age.

In addition to societal costs, research studies indicate substance misuse can have many health and personal consequences for individuals (USDHHS 2016). The direct effects depend on the specific substances used, how much and how often they are used, how they are taken (e.g., orally vs. injected), and other factors. Acute effects often range from changes in mood and basic body functions, such as heart rate or blood pressure, to overdose and death. Alcohol misuse and drug use can also have long-term effects on physical and mental health and can lead to substance use disorders. Drug use is associated with chronic pain conditions and cardiovascular and cardiopulmonary diseases. Alcohol misuse is associated with liver and pancreatic diseases, hypertension, reproductive system disorders, trauma, stroke, and a variety of cancers, including cancer of the oral cavity, esophagus, larynx, pharynx, liver, colon, and rectum. Substance misuse also can affect nutrition and sleep and increase the risk for trauma, violence, injury, and contraction of communicable diseases, such as HIV/AIDS and Hepatitis C.

Within the United States population specifically, the elderly are acknowledged as a sub-population increasingly vulnerable to substance use, misuse, and abuse issues. One study has noted that while data indicates "older adults have not demonstrated high rates of alcohol or other drug us compared with younger adults. These facts have helped perpetuate a misconception that older adults do not use or abuse mood-altering substances" (Kuerbis et al. 2014, 1). The authors further assert that "Indeed, substantial evidence suggests that substance use among older adults has been under-identified for decades. The aging of the baby boom generation creates a new urgency to effectively identify and treat substance use among older adults." (Kuerbis et al. 2014, 1). The authors cite extensive data on high prevalence rates of SUD specifically among baby boomers as they age, noting that "SUD rates among people older than 50 years are projected to increase from about 2.8 million in 2006 to 5.7 million in 2020" (Kuerbis et al. 2014, 1). Other researchers have supported these concerns and have additionally a concern specifically for abuse of opioids and other prescription drugs, noting that "….as the 'baby boom' cohort ages, it appears likely that the proportion of older adults using these drugs and experiencing substance abuse associated problems will also increase" (Kalapatapu and Sullivan 2010, 3).

Medicare beneficiaries appear particularly vulnerable to substance abuse use, misuse and SUD, given that an estimated 95% of all Americans aged 65 years and older are Medicare beneficiaries (Mather et al. 2015). However, the Substance Abuse and Mental Health Services SAMHSA that in 2016 Medicare represented only the fourth largest payer for treatment of persons with mental and/or substance use disorders (M/SUDs), or only 13% of all national health spending on M/SUDs (SAMHSA 2019a). SAMHSA does not report SUD only data separate from the M/SUD data.

In 2018, there were approximately 5.1 million Medicare beneficiaries served under Medicare home health, or about 10% of all Medicare beneficiaries (Centers for Medicare & Medicaid Services [CMMS] 2018; Mather et al. 2015). CMS data appears to indicate limited focus on substance use, misuse, and SUD in the Medicare home health program. For example, using CMS 2016 Medicare Beneficiary Survey data, Avalere Health (2018) found no SUD, substance use, substance misuse, mental health, or M/SUD diagnosis among the top twenty primary International Classification of Diseases, Version 10 (ICD-10) diagnosis, which represented 58% of all 2017 Medicare home health claims. Ironically, mental health is a significant issue for Medicare beneficiaries with CMS reporting in 2015 44% of all Medicare home health beneficiaries had a severe mental illness (SMI), which is defined "as having depression or other mental disorder including bipolar disorder, schizophrenia, and other psychoses." (Avalere Health 2018, 28) The SMI data is limited because it only includes severe mental illness and because CMS data does not even capture data on substance use, misuse, or SUD, either in the aggregate or by type of substance; not even as a subset of its data on mental health conditions (Avalere Health 2018).

BACKGROUND

The limited insight from government data on the prevalence and coverage of substance misuse, use and SUD in Medicare home health prompted a literature review on studies of the topic.

The literature review used Cinahl, PubMed, Medline, Cochrane Library, Campbell Collaboration, PsycINFO, Sociological Abstracts, and Social Science Abstracts databases with an search period of January 1, 1965 through September 30, 2012 followed by an updated search after the study was conducted covering October 1, 2012 through June 30, 2019. Multiple keywords were used in the search: substance use and home care; substance abuse and home care; opioid use and home care; home care social work; Medicare home health social work; psycho-social care and Medicare home health; and substance use and abuse and the elderly. The searches yielded multiple studies on home health, home health social work, home health nursing and generally on substance use and abuse among the elderly but no studies specifically on prevalence, coverage, or consequences of substance use or abuse in the Medicare home health setting.

The present study was designed to address this gap in the existing literature regarding the topic. The study presents the results of an exploratory, qualitative design using semi-structured interviews of 26 home care social workers in the New York City metropolitan area between January 2013 and May 2014. The study used interviews to probe social workers' perceptions of the nature and extent of substance use and abuse prevalence and coverage in Medicare home health and the impact on patients, caregivers, and Medicare.

METHODS

The study used a grounded theory approach (Corbin and Strauss 2007). Grounded theory is the research methodology of choice because it was developed for interpreting qualitative data in the absence of a pre-existing theory. In the present study, the existing literature does not provide insight into how home care nurses perceive the coverage of SDOH and the impact on patients, caregivers, and payers, including Medicare. Data were collected through interviews of 37 home care nurses, selected from the New York City metropolitan area between January 2013 and May 2014. Participants were selected using a snowball convenience sampling technique, whereby home care industry professionals known to the author identified potential interviewees. In-person interviews were conducted at locations convenient to participants and off-site from where they worked. An interview guide was used to help standardize the data collection, and all participants were assured of anonymity and confidentiality through an informed consent form they signed. Qualitative analysis began shortly after the initial data were collected and resulted in additional questions and probes that were applied to subsequent interviews, in an ongoing iterative process. Analysis followed the grounded theory three-stage coding of interview data: open, axial, and selective coding.

Open coding was used to fracture the data to "identify some categories, their properties, and dimensional locations" (Corbin and Strauss 2007, 97). The coding and classification generated a list of 268 codes. Code and category labels were created, systematically sorted, compared, and contrasted until they were complete, with no new codes or categories produced and all data accounted for. Through axial coding, multiple phenomena were identified from the connected categories and subcategories. These phenomena included the Medicare decision-making framework, home care nurse perceptions of substance use and abuse, home care nurse perceptions of ability to address substance use and abuse in care planning and delivery, and home care nurse perceptions of impacts of ignoring substance use and abuse issues. Finally, using selective coding, a "story line" was identified and a "story" written that integrated the axial coding phenomena (Corbin and Strauss 2007). The story that emerged was the influence of Medicare home health's lack of coverage of substance use and abuse on patients, caregivers, and payers.

In keeping with the grounded theory approach, the data analysis and interpretation were facilitated by analytical and self-reflective memo writing, which helped move empirical data to a conceptual level; expanded and refined the data and codes; developed core categories and interrelationships; and integrated the experiences, interactions, and processes embodied in the data (Corbin and Strauss 2007). All initial abstraction, analysis, and interpretation were done by the author of this article. After the initial process, all abstraction, analysis, and interpretations were reviewed by two additional experienced qualitative researchers, each of whom had a doctoral degree in social work and more than fifteen years' experience doing government-funded qualitative research on substance abuse. Any differences were discussed by the two external reviewers and the author to reach final decisions used for the study results. All analyses were done using ATLAS.ti software.

Social workers were selected for the study because they are the only professionals covered under the Medicare home health benefit who are trained to conduct psychosocial interventions, including substance use disorders. A 2019 study by the National Academies of Science, Engineering, and Medicine (NASEM 2019) further emphasized the need to integrate more social care, delivered by social workers, at all levels in the health delivery system to better address substance use and mental health conditions. There also is significant literature on the effectiveness of social workers addressing social work in multiple health care settings for substance use and mental health conditions (Berrett-Abebe et al. 2020; Rizzo and Rowe 2016; Rizzo et al. 2016; Rowe et al. 2017; Rowe et al. 2019).

Table 1. Social worker participant demographic characteristics

Characteristic	Number	Percent
Gender		
Male	2	5%
Female	35	95%
Race/Ethnicity		
Caucasian, Non-Hispanic	30	81%
Hispanic	3	8%
African American	2	5%
Asian American	1	3%
Other	1	3%
Age Range		
> 55	2	5%
45-55	28	76%
36-44	4	11%
25-35	3	8%
Years as a Home Care Nurse		
> 10	3	8%
6-10	28	76%
1-5	5	13%
< 1	1	3%
Average Patient Caseload		
26-30	1	3%
20-25	32	86%
< 20	4	11%

Limited demographic data was collected from study participants using a short survey. The results appear in Table 1. Overall the social workers were

45-55 years old (76%); female (95%); had 6-10 years of home care experience (76%); and had an average caseload of 20-25 patients (86%). Statistical analysis of the demographic variables' impact on study outcomes was not done due to the qualitative nature of the study.

RESULTS

Five themes emerged from the interviews, which are detailed below with supporting quotes.

High Frequency of Substance Use, Abuse, and SUD: "They are Like Ghosts Haunting Us"

"It is as common as heart disease or cancer but we simply act like it is not there," according to social worker QT. All social workers interviewed (100%) agreed there is a high frequency of substance use, misuse, and SUD among their patients:

> "It hangs over us all the time. Medicare doesn't cover it, but it's there. It's almost like a ghost haunting us, hanging over us while we try to ignore it and treat what we are paid for like healing wounds, diabetes, heart and respiratory conditions mainly." (Social Worker HG)
>
> "I have been doing home care for about 18 years. Substance problems are very common/. Medication management works for some but many are non-compliant and it is more than simply taking meds. There are underlying social and environmental issues. I'd say 75% of our patients have serious drug abuse issues." (Social Worker EH)
>
> "Substance abuse is our most consistent issue across all patients. We never do not use it as a diagnosis. Our patients all have a primary diagnosis that relates to an acute physical health need; not mental health or substance use. But in reality they all have a substance abuse or misuse issue." (Social Worker PS)

"If you include alcohol abuse, I'd say 80 to 90% of our patients have a substance abuse issue. That is not counting their caregivers, who we can't treat anyway. Many of them [the caregivers] have SUD issues too." (Social Worker SH)

Failure to Professionally Assess and Treat Substance Use Issues

"Patient substance use behaviors are not assessed and infrequently treated by a trained professional," according to social worker TC. Social workers were concerned that neither Medicare nor their agencies require assessment and treatment of SUD and other substance issues, let alone mandating evidence-based assessment measures and treatments. Ninety-five percent of social workers interviewed believed there was no professional assessment or treatment of substance use, misuse, or abuse:

"I find it absurd. Substance abuse issues exist, often all over the [medical] record, but we can't professionally assess or treat it. There are evidence-based interventions and assessment tools. I learned about them in graduate school and continuing education courses, but we can't use them. Isn't that ridiculous? Why can't we? I ask it all the time. I am told it's not required on the OASIS [Outcome and Assessment Information Set] and that it is a chronic condition, which we are not allowed to treat. We focus on acute episodes. Drug abuse is considered chronic. Medicare won't pay for it at home. It makes no sense to me." (Social Worker TJ)

"Our agency has no policy and procedure protocol for assessing and treating substance use." (Social Worker DG)

"Medicare seems so outdated. We have many patients on meds, increasingly many on opioids for pain, and we can't treat them. It's all over the news. There is an opiod epidemic Things like naloxone are being offered outside home care, but not for our patients who are homebound. They are such desparate souls and we can't do anything for them. It is so sad." (Social Worker TS)

Lack of Coverage of Substance Misuse and SUD Exacerbates Physical Health, Mental Health, and Substance Use Issues

"We do not assess or treat substance issues. That complicates most conditions, especially heart and respiratory conditions and things like depression. It makes anyone with drug issues even worse," said social worker MS. All social workers (100%) agreed that the inability to cover substance abuse issues contributed to exacerbation of existing physical and mental health conditions:

> "You asked for an example. I'll give you one. A patient comes in diabetes. We focus on the immediate situation, the diabetes issue; that's it. So, I'm thinking of several cases like this. And in many cases they are alcoholics or on heavy duty opioids for pain to deal with pain. The drug problem limits their compliance." (Social Worker SF)
>
> "I have an example. I had a patient who had limited mobility due COPD with diabetes comorbidity. They also were depressed. Surprise! What do people do when they are depressed? A lot of our patients drink and take ills which numbs them for a bit and then makes them worse, physically and mentally. That is what this patient did." (Social Worker RA)

Inability to Provide Transportation and Personal Care Assistants Limits Patients Ability to Get Outpatient Substance Treatment Services: "It's a Downright Shame"

Most nurses (95%) expressed frustration with their inability to facilitate patients obtaining substance misuse and SUD in Medicare-covered outpatient settings:

> "The closest place to get [substance use and SUD] help is an outpatient clinic. Our patients are homebound. They can't get there easily. If they could they would not be on home care. So what do we do? We give no care at home and no assistance to get the outpatient care." (Social Worker YU)

"I have had a lot of patients with drug issues; so have my colleagues. Most of it is caused, ironically, by the medications they take for their [physical health] condition. There are others who just are chronic alcoholics or drug users because of their life experiences. So, here they are being homebound, which is required for Medicare home health eligibility. They need a lot of help with daily activities. We can't do much for that since we have limited use of home health aides. Then, on top of it, for many, there are drug issues, which we are not allowed to treat. Medicare won't cover it. So they need to go to an outpatient program. That sounds reasonable, right? NO. Many are so homebound they need considerable assistance. Medicare won't cover it so unless you have significant money, you can't go." (Social Worker PC)

Failure to Address Substance Use Issues Contribute to Home Care Readmissions, Re-Hospitalizations, and Caregiver Burden: "It's Your Worst Nightmare"

CMS does not measure or track re-admissions to home care, let alone by reason. However, nurses indicated failure to acknowledge, assess, and treat SUD and related substance issues results in a continual stream of home care re-admissions, re-hospitalizations, and increased caregiver burden. All **social workers** (100%) believed the inability to assess and treat substance misuse issues, including SUD, contributes to home care readmissions, re-hospitalizations, and increased caregiver burden:

"We readmit a lot [of patients]. Most that we readmit return to us in 30-60 days after discharge. I think a lot of why they return is because they have no one at home to help with post-discharge follow-up. Everything falls apart. Sometimes they have a competent caregiver but many have caregivers who have their own issues, including drug issues, and we cannot touch that. We can't treat the caregivers. I'd get fired if I did that. Medicare doesn't cover it so the agency wouldn't get reimbursed. But it would help everyone and probably reduce those costly re-admissions everyone complains about." (Social Worker RM)

"I am a social worker. I know a drug issue affects both your physical and mental health. We learn that it is not unusual for some [patient physical] health issues to result in substance abuse or vice versa. We are taught this. Medicare doesn't care. What's the result? We get frustrated and watch patients get worse. We discharge patients and they return. I'd say it's the norm; about a third of the patients. What's the point? Medicare complains about costs and here they do not let us treat a major source of costs: substance abuse. It is so frustrating." Social Worker ST

LIMITATIONS

The study was a qualitative, exploratory study. As such it does not address causality and has several limitations including: small sample size; lack of random sampling for sample selection; and lack of a randomized controlled trial experimental design to test specific interventions against a control group.

CONCLUSION

Despite its limitations, the study does begin to address a gap in the literature and policy by exploring nurse perceptions of the prevalence and impact of lack of assessment, coverage, and treatment of substance use and abuse on Medicare home health patients and their caregivers. The study supports other studies on the current and projected increase of substance use and SUD among the elderly (Kalapataku and Sullivan 2010; Kueribis et al. 2014; Mather et al. 2015), adding qualitative insight to its occurrence in the Medicare home health setting. The story told in the nurse interviews also identifies some specific areas for potential policy reform to benefit patients, home health professionals, and the Medicare program. The initiation of the new Medicare Home Health Patient-Driven Groupings Model (PDGM) in 2020 provides a timely opportunity for such reforms (Abt Associates and CMMS 2019).

Contrary to the home health social worker interviews and studies on substance abuse among the elderly, Medicare does not publicly report on SUD or substance abuse among home health beneficiaries. For example there was no substance use code listed among the top 20 Primary International Classification of Diseases, Version 10 (ICD-10) Diagnoses for All Home Health Claims (Avalere Health 2018). These top twenty diagnoses represented 58% of all claims. In addition, neither SUD nor substance abuse are listed in Medicare's reporting on severe mental illness (Avalere Health 2018). Medicare does not report such data because it fails to capture the data. The OASIS currently has no section requiring nurses to assess, or otherwise measure, the existence of substance abuse or risk level for abuse at either admission, recertification, or discharge (CMMS 2019b). This contrasts with Medicare requiring nurses complete the PHQ-2, an evidence-based depression scale (Kroenke et al. 2003), on the OASIS. The result is Medicare publicly reporting data that indicates 44% of all Medicare home health beneficiaries in 2015 had a severe mental illness (SMI) and 94% of those with an SMI had depression (Avalere Health 2018). A remedy for the lack of home health beneficiary substance abuse data would be for CMS to add a mandated, evidence-based substance use assessment section to the current OASIS with a requirement that patients scoring as having SUD or a specified significant risk of abuse level must receive treatment. SAMHSA has developed multiple evidence-based assessment tools which are used in inpatient and outpatient programs which Medicare could adopt to systematically measure and report on substance abuse in home health (SAMHSA 2019b).

However, improved assessment and reporting requirements do not guarantee that patients assessed or at risk of substance abuse will receive treatment. Medicare currently covers mental health and substance abuse services in inpatient, outpatient and partial hospitalization programs but not in home health (Center for Medicare Advocacy 2019a; Medicare Benefit Policy Manual). The only exception is the possible use of a psychiatric nurse in Medicare home health which "would only be considered medically reasonable and necessary if the evidence demonstrates that the patient is in danger to self or others" (Center for Medicare Advocacy 2019a) and assuming a psychiatric nurse is available. To ensure professional treatment of home health patients assessed with or at-risk of substance abuse, Medicare would have to mandate that patients receive treatment and modify coverage and reimbursement rules to include such treatments. SAMHSA has developed multiple evidence-based treatments which are used in inpatient and outpatient programs which Medicare could adopt to systematically measure and report on substance abuse in home health (SAMHSA 2019b). Expansion of the current Medicare home health social work benefit might be the most feasible avenue to provide such care. Currently the home health social work benefit is limited to only a few individual psycho-social therapy visits, no family therapy and no group therapy (Cabin 2019b; Medicare Benefits Manual). Payment for such services would need to be accommodated within the new PDGM system or as a specified, separately reimbursement add-on payment. The covered mandated treatments also would enable Medicare to track progress of patients and possibly include such data in its home health quality improvement reporting (Centers for Medicare and Medicaid Services 2019a).

In addition to reforms creating meaningful assessment and treatment of Medicare home health patients with substance use issues at home, Medicare could also facilitate homebound Medicare patients' ability to receive outpatient substance abuse services. This could be done by Medicare covering costs of transportation and accompanying personal care assistants to facilitate homebound Medicare home health patient access to covered outpatient substance abuse services. The PDGM system would require a coverage and payment change to facilitate such services. However, Congress and CMS already have set a precedent for coverage of such services through Medicare Advantage plans (Cabin 2019a).

These reforms seem reasonable for Congress and CMS consideration given the current and projected data on SUD and substance abuse among the elderly. They also seem reasonable because both Congress and CMS have recently recognized the relevance of social determinants of health and have begun efforts to cover transportation, personal care assistants, and other social needs services to improve patient outcomes and reduce Medicare costs (Cabin 2019b). The move toward focusing on social determinants expands home-based care beyond the current Medicare home health model, allowing a greater focus on factors associated with substance use and mental health conditions. As a result, a significant expansion of the Medicare home health social work benefit and requirements for SUD assessment, treatment, and public reporting seem worthy of Congressional action, particularly given CMS' recent recognition of the value of such an approach and the current and projected prevalence of substance use among the elderly.

References

Abt Associates and Centers for Medicare and Medicaid Services. (2019). *Centers for Medicare and Medicaid Services Patient-Drive Groupings Model.* Retrieved from: https://www.cms.gov/Outreach-and-Education/Outreach/NPC/National-Prover-Calls-and-Events-Items/2019-02-12-PDGM.htmll .

Avalere Health. Home Health Chartbook 2018: *Prepared for the Alliance for Home Health Quality and Innovation.* ahhqi.org/images/uploads/AHHQI_2018_Chartbook_09.21.2018.pdf. Published September 2018. Accessed August 20, 2019.

Berrett-Abebe, J., Donelan, K., Berkman, B., Auerbach, D. & Maramaldi, P. (2020). Physician and nurse practitioner perceptions of social worker and community health worker roles in primary care practices caring for frail elders: Insights for social work. *Social Work in Health Care*, *59*(1), 46-60.

Cabin, W. (2019a). Home Care Nurses Claim Medicare Ignores Social Determinants of Health. *Home Health Care Management & Practice, 31* (4), 224-230.

Cabin, W. (2019b). *Medicare Home Care Increases Health Risks by Ignoring Patient Social Work Needs*. Unpublished.

Center for Medicare Advocacy. (2019a). *Medicare Coverage of Mental Health and Substance Abuse Services*. Retrieved from: https://www.medicareadvocacy.org/medicare-info/medicare-coverage-of-mental-health-services/.

Center for Medicare Advocacy. (2019b). *Home Health Care*. Retrieved from: https://www.medicareadvocacy.org/medicare-info/home-health-care.

Centers for Medicare and Medicaid Services. (2019a). *Home Health Quality Reporting Program*. Retrieved from: https://www.cms.gov/Medicare/Quality-Initiatives-Patient-Assessment-Instruments/HomeHealthQualityInits/index.html.

Centers for Medicare and Medicare Services. (2019b). *Medicare Coverage of Substance Abuse Services*. MLN Matters Number: SE 1604. April 28, 2016. Department of Health and Human Services. Centers for Medicare and Medicaid Services.

Corbin, J. & Strauss, A. (2007). *Basics of Qualitative Research: Techniques and Procedures for Developing Grounded Theory*. Thousand Oaks, CA: SAGE.

Kalapatapu, R. K. & Sullivan, M. A. (2010). Prescription Use Disorders in Older Adults. *American Journal of Addiction*, *19*(6), 515-522.

Kroenke, K., Spitzer, R. I. & Williams, J. B. (2003). The Patient Health questionnaire-2: validity of a two-item depression screener. *Med. Care*, *41*, 1284-1292.

Kuerbis, A., Sacco, P., Blazer, D. G. & Moore, A. A. (2014). Substance Use Among Older Adults. *Clin Geriatr Med*, *30*(3), 629–654.

Mather, M., Jacobsen, L. A. & Pollard, K. M. (2015). Aging in the United States, *Population Bulletin*, *70*(2).

Medicare Benefit Policy Manual, Chapter 7, *Home Health Services*. Retrieved from https://www.cms.gov/Regulations-and-Guidance/Guidance/Manuals/.../bp102c07.pdf.

Medicare Payment Advisory Commission. (2018a). *Medicare Basics: Home Health Services*. Washington, DC: Author.

Medicare Payment Advisory Commission. (2018b). *Report to Congress: Medicare Payment Policy*, Chapter 9. Washington, DC: Author.

National Academies of Science, Engineering and Medicine. (2019). *Integrating Social Care Into The Delivery of Health Care: Moving Upstream to Improve the Nation's Health*. Washington, DC: National Academies Press.

Rizzo, V. M. & Rowe, J. M. (2016). Cost Effectiveness of Social work services in Aging: An Updated Systematic Review. *Research on Social Work Practice*, *26*(6), 653-667.

Rizzo, V. M., Rowe, J. M., Kricke, G. S., Krajci, K. & Golden, R. (2016). AIMS: A Care Coordination Model to Improve Patient Outcomes. *Health and Social Work*, *41*(3), 191-195.

Rowe, J., Rizzo, V. M., Guthrie, D., Vail, M. R., Kang, S. K. & Golden, R. (2019). The Electronic Health record: Documenting the Unique Contributions of Social Workers. *Health and Social Work*, *44*(2), 123-128.

Rowe, J. M., Rizzo, V. M., Vail, M. R., Kang, S. K. & Golden, R. (2017). The role of social workers in addressing nonmedical needs in primary health care. *Social Work in Health Care*, *56*(6), 435-449.

Substance Abuse and Mental Health Services Administration. (2014). *Projections of National Expenditures for Treatment of Mental Health and Substance Use Disorders, 2010-2020.* HHS Publication No. SMA-14-4883. Rockville, MD: Author.

Substance Abuse and Mental Health Services Administration. (2019a). *Evidence-based Practices Resource Center*. Retrieved from: https://www.samhsa.gov/ebp-resource-center.

Substance Abuse and Mental Health Services Administration. (2019b). *Screening Tools*. Retrieved from: https://www.integration.samhsa.gov/clinical-practice/screening-tools.

U.S. Department of Health and Human Services (HHS), Office of the Surgeon General. (2016). *Facing Addiction in America: The Surgeon General's Report on Alcohol, Drugs, and Health*. Washington, DC: Author.

U.S. Department of Health and Human Services (HHS), Office of the Surgeon General. (2018). *Facing Addiction in America: The Surgeon General's Spotlight on Opioids*. Washington, DC: Author.

Whiteford, H. A., Degenhardt, L., Rehm, J., Baxter, A. J., Ferrari, A. J., Erskine, H. E. & Vos, T. (2013). Global burden of disease attributable to mental and substance use disorders: Findings from the Global Burden of Disease Study 2010. *The Lancet*, *382*(9904), 1575-1586.

In: Elderly Care
Editor: Sean M. Eckstein

ISBN: 978-1-53618-446-4

Chapter 9

"I LOVE WHAT I DO" HOW TO SUPPORT HOME CARE AIDES IN DOING THE WORK THEY LOVE

Sandra S. Butler*
School of Social Work, University of Maine, Orono, Maine

ABSTRACT

As our population ages and older adults needing assistance increasingly prefer to say in their homes, the demand for home care aides (HCAs) is growing dramatically. Currently demand for these valuable workers far outweighs supply. It is imperative that we improve job conditions in order to maintain current workers and attract new ones. This chapter will review findings from two studies concerning HCAs in the rural state of Maine. The first, a mixed-method, longitudinal inquiry (n = 261), carried out from 2008 to 2010, examined factors contributing to job turnover for HCAs. Findings indicated that many workers left their home care jobs despite loving the work and feeling very committed to their clients; more than one third of the sample (n = 90) terminated over the 18 months of data collection. Low compensation, lack of benefits, irregular

* Corresponding Author's Email: sbutler@maine.edu.

hours, and worker burnout contributed to turnover decisions according to study participants. A more recent in-depth qualitative study examined the structural and psychological components of the HCA job that influence a worker's feeling of empowerment. This inquiry (n = 8; 2018) revealed the deep connections research participants felt with their work and their clients, while simultaneously struggling with challenges such as poor wages, uneven support from agencies, minimal training, and not being adequately valued in the larger health care team. This chapter discusses the findings from both these studies and, from the perspective of the study participants, offer recommendations for improving job conditions so as to make recruitment of new workers easier and retention of current workers more likely.

INTRODUCTION

Home care aides (HCAs) provide assistance to people with chronic diseases and functional impairments who wish to remain in their homes—and most do want to remain at home. Currently in the United States (US), as is true in most developed countries, there is a greater demand for these workers than there is supply. This chapter examines the job experience of HCAs based on two studies in the state of Maine that provided workers the opportunity to describe the work they do in their own words. It provides recommendations for improving job conditions in order to increase both recruitment and retention.

A JOB IN HIGH DEMAND

Home care aides provide help to individuals who need assistance with activities of daily living (such as bathing and dressing) and instrumental activities of daily living (such as cooking and cleaning). Most people receive that assistance from informal caregivers, i.e., family and friends. The need for paid caregivers, or formal caregivers, has increased with changes in the workforce and in the structure of families: more women work outside the home than was true in past generations; simultaneously, there has been an increase in divorce rates and a decline in the number of children families have (Hess & Hegewisch 2019). As informal caregivers are less available, or not available at all, HCAs pick up this crucial caring work.

Currently, about 8 million Americans who need personal assistance live at home, and 15 percent of those individuals require paid HCAs (Iezzoni, Gallopyn & Scales 2019). The need for personal assistance services is expected to grow in tandem with the aging of the US population. The number of Americans adults aged 65 and older is projected to double between 2015 and 2060 (from 46 to 98 million) and for those, aged 85 and older, this increase will be more than three-fold (from 6 to 20 million; Hess & Hegwisch 2019).

Not surprisingly, the HCA workforce in the US has also been growing. It more than doubled between 2008 and 2018, increasing in size from 898,000 to 2.3 million workers (Scales 2019). This is likely an undercount as these numbers do not include workers employed privately by individuals needing assistance, but only those employed through agencies. The workforce is expected to add another million jobs between 2018 and 2028, making it the US occupation with the greatest projected growth (Scales 2019). Like most caring professions, HCA jobs are predominantly filled by women (87% in 2017). Moreover, based on 2017 data, 62 percent of HCAs are people of color and 31 percent were born outside the US. While one in five have an Associate's degree or higher, more than half have a high school degree or less in 2017 (Scales 2019). While home health aides employed by Medicare-certified home health agencies are required to have at least 75 hours of training, leading to the certified nursing assistant (CNA) title, there are no federal training requirements for personal care aides—the focus of this chapter. States are free to develop their own training requirements for HCAs, but not all do (Scales 2019); Maine requires its personal care aides to have 50 hours of training.

Challenges of the HCA Job

There are many rewarding aspects of the HCA job as will be detailed later in this chapter, and which have been identified in other studies (e.g.,

Stacey 2011). But the challenges often outweigh the rewards leading to high rates of turnover, estimated to range from 40 to 60 percent annually. A study in 2018 found worker turnover to have reached a historic 82 percent among home care agencies (Scales 2019), indicating the crisis situation we are currently facing. There are an array of hazards that can affect the safety and health of home care aides. These include musculoskeletal issues related to lifting and transferring clients, risks involved with physically demanding housekeeping, and hazards related to transportation and negotiating snow- and ice-covered entrances to homes (Seavey& Marquand 2011; Stacey 2011). Emotional stressors also play into the nature of this work including having too much responsibility with inadequate training, dealing with deterioration and death of their clients, or working within bureaucratic rules that do not always jibe with what workers believe is in the best interest of their clients (Stacey 2011).

Low compensation is a key challenge in attracting and keeping HCAs in this important work. The median hourly wage for personal care aides in 2018 was $11.40. Moreover more than one third of home care workers (38%) did not have full-time employment in that year (Scales 2019). Despite working in the healthcare field, 16 percent of home care workers lacked health insurance in 2017; of those who did have health insurance, 42 percent were covered by Medicaid. Employer coverage was not available for many due part-time hours or prohibitive costs (Scales 2019). The combination of low wages and part-time hours results in many HCAs living in poverty; nearly one in two (48%) lived below 200 percent of the federal poverty line in 2017. More than half (53%) received some form of public assistance (Scales 2019).

Ultimately turnover among home care workers harms the three "key stakeholders" (Dawson & Surpin 2001) of long-term care: consumers and their families; providers (i.e., home care agencies and companies); and the workers themselves. High rates of turnover mean consumers will have inconsistent care; providers will bear the cost of increased recruitment and orientation; and workers who remain will need to fill in extra, unplanned shifts potentially causing increased stress and injuries (Dawson & Surpin 2001). The two studies described below sought to understand the rewards and challenges HCAs experience on their jobs and factors that might lead them to leave their jobs.

HOME CARE WORKER RETENTION STUDY (HCWRS)-2008-2010

The HCWRS, funded by the National Institute on Aging, was implemented to examine factors predicting turnover and retention among HCAs in Maine, and to understand more about how these workers experience their jobs. The study involved two mail surveys and one telephone interview with a sample of 261 HCAs drawn from 11 Maine home care agencies. These 11 agencies covered all regions of the state with study participants living in each of the 16 counties. Once agreeing to participate in the study, agencies sent a mail survey instrument (Time 1) to all their HCAs (n = 496) in October 2008; over half of the workers completed the survey (n = 261), giving a response rate of 52.6%. Participating agencies provided the study team with regular reports of study participant terminations during the 18 months after completion of the first survey. Workers who left their employment received a second mail survey and completed a telephone interview lasting between 15 and 30 minutes soon after their termination (n = 90); workers who remained employed throughout the 18-month study period (n = 171) received the second survey and completed the telephone interview during the spring and summer of 2010 (Time 2). Study participants received $20 grocery gift cards at both Time 1 and Time 2.

The Time 1 survey instrument assessed demographic information and current home care jobs, and included several standardized scales measuring health status and job experience factors such as job satisfaction, burnout, and empowerment. These job experience measures were also included in the shorter Time 2 survey instrument, which study participants completed after they had either terminated their employment or at the end of the data collection period, if they remained employed. The telephone interview was composed of 18 open-ended questions covering topics such as why they had left, if terminated, or what might make them consider leaving, if still employed; what aspects of their HCA work brought them satisfaction; what parts of the job they found draining; and their views of their employing home care agency.

Sample Description

Study participants ranged in age from 19 to 82 with an average age of 46. The vast majority was female (94.6%), and most study participants identified as White (93.5%). Twenty-nine study participants (11.1%) said they were Franco-American, three identified as Latinx(1.1%), and nine (3.4%) were born outside the U.S. While similar to the national demographics of the home care workforce in terms of age and gender, the Maine sample was disproportionately White and U.S. born, reflecting the composition of the general Maine population (US Census Bureau 2010). Over a quarter of the study participants lacked any type of health insurance (28.0%); a similar number (28.7%) received Medicaid, 8.4% received Medicare, and only 14 (5.4%) study participants received health insurance through their home care agency.

Job tenure at the home care agency through which study participants had received the survey ranged from "just started" to over 12 years, with a mean tenure of 2.6 years. Hourly wages were low, ranging from $7.50 to $13.50 with an average wage of $9.05. Study participants reported working from no hours in the preceding four weeks to 504 hours, with an average of 18.0 hours per week, and driving from 0 to 1,750 unreimbursed miles in the preceding four weeks, with an average of 46.1 unreimbursed miles per week.

Findings

Quantitative analysis, using logistic regression, revealed four factors that significantly predicted turnover in this sample: younger age; not having health insurance; lower mental health scores (i.e., higher levels of depression and anxiety); and, surprisingly, higher scores on a scale measuring personal accomplishment that was part of a larger scale measuring job burnout. As the focus of this chapter is the qualitative analysis of study participant interviews, I refer the reader to an earlier article reporting on this study for a more in-depth description of measures, data analysis, and discussion of the findings related to turnover (see Butler, Wardamasky & Brennan-Ing 2012).

Of the 90 study participants who terminated during the study period, 88 (97.8%) completed telephone interviews soon after they left their jobs. Reasons for leaving fell into three broad categories: 1) that the job did not seem worthwhile given low wages, inconsistent hours, and unreimbursed mileage; 2) personal reasons, such as health, retirement, or family needs; and 3) burnout caused by poor communication with agency, difficult clients or client family members, or having clients die (Butler, Simpson & Brennan 2010).

Under the theme "*Job Not Worthwhile,*" lack of compensation emerged as a primary concern, as stated by a 41-year-old female study participant: "The pay wasn't that great. The part where they didn't pay the mileage. I ended up losing money on the whole thing so it really wasn't worth it for me." The theme, *"Personal Reasons,"* was composed of study participant situations that led them to terminate that were not related to their perceptions of their jobs. For example, the oldest study participant said, "Well I'm 84 years old, so it's probably time that I did stop." Another study participant in her 40s was told she needed to stop the work, which can be both physically and emotionally demanding. She said:

> I have herniated disks. My doctor called up and said "you're all done" and I'm like what? I've been doing this for… I started when I was 18 and I'm over 41 now. I mean that was a long time being in the health care field. Seeing all that and then to be told that I can't do that anymore, that was like a huge blow.

While burnout was not a predictor of turnover in the quantitative analysis in this study, it did emerge as an important theme in the qualitative analysis. For example, a 25-year-old study participant described her mounting stress from work with a home care agency:

> The constant lack of communication. Never really knowing what was going on. That caused me a lot of stress. I am a planner. I have things set-up and that's the way I expect them to go and things were never the way they said they were going to go. And, it just kind of had me in a tailspin, stressed out.

Another example under the "*Burnout*," theme came from a 27-year-old who described how working with sick and dying individuals could take its toll:

> When my long-term client passed away, I actually ended up on Valium, because I had such anxiety. I don't think they give you enough warning before going into hospice. I went in and got really attached with this woman. She was absolutely amazing and it took a huge toll, which I didn't expect it to.

Further analysis of the narrative data from study participants who had terminated examined responses to questions that specifically asked them what they found satisfying about their work and what they found draining (Butler, Wardamaski & Brennan-Ing 2012). Study participants also described aspects of the job they found rewarding or challenging in response to other questions in the interview as well (e.g., questions regarding relationships with their clients and employers). The rewarding components that were reported included the appreciation they felt from clients; the personal satisfaction of helping clients be able to remain in their homes; the autonomy of being one's own boss; the flexibility of hours; and, for some, the relief of loneliness in their own lives. Challenging components included low pay, lack of sick leave or paid time off, death of clients, difficult client behaviors, poor communication with home care agency/company, not enough or inconsistent hours, and unreimbursed mileage. Among the 88 study participants who terminated their employment and completed interviews, 47 (53.4%) reported more rewarding experiences than challenging ones, 37 (42.0%) reported more challenging aspects to their job than rewarding ones, and 4 (4.5%) reported an equal number of rewarding and challenging components to the work.

The HCWRS revealed that workers generally found considerable satisfaction in their home care jobs, but there were a number of components of the work that could cause them to leave the profession for jobs with more consistent hours, higher pay, less emotional stress, and more supervisor support. In the years since the HCWRS was completed, the need for HCAs has only grown. Legislative changes in Maine have led to small increases in wages (though both targeted raises for HCAs and a more general increase in the State minimum wage). Nonetheless, home care agencies continue to report difficulties in recruitment and retention in the current tight labor market. In 2018, as part of a two-state pilot inquiry on how home care workers experience empowerment, I interviewed eight HCAs in Maine; findings from that study are presented next.

2018 HCA Job Experience Study

The eight study participants were recruited through flyers at agencies and word of mouth. They were all women, White, and born in the US. The ranged in age from 20 to 64 and had been working in the field anywhere from two weeks to 34 years, with an average of 8.4 years. One of the study participants worked privately and the other seven worked for three different statewide for-profit, home care agencies. Four interviews were completed in person and four took place by telephone. The interview questions asked study participants about: 1) structural aspects of their job, such as whether they had the information, resources and support they needed and if there were opportunities for advancement; and 2) psychological aspects of the job, such as their feelings of competence, level of autonomy, whether they felt that they were making an impact, and how meaningful the work was for them.

Findings

In terms of the psychological aspects of the job, all eight study participants found the work meaningful and thought they positively impacted their clients' lives. Moreover, they enjoyed the autonomy of the work and perceived themselves as competent. Their responses were more mixed in terms of the structural components of their work. Some were satisfied with the level of support they received from their supervisors and felt they had the resources and information they needed to carry out their jobs. Others identified deficiencies in all three of these areas. While a few thought there were some opportunities for advancement, if one had the time, money and/or inclination, others described the work as rather dead-end. In general, the eight study participants fell into three categories: "*Satisfied with Job,*" (n = 3), "*It Works, But We Need More Support,*" (n = 3), and "*On My Way Out,*" (n = 2; Butler 2020).

One study participant, who fell into the "*Satisfied with Job*" category, was a 60-year-old HCA who worked 65 hours each week across two agencies. She had been with her primary agency for nine years, received health insurance through her employment, and found great satisfaction in her job: "I love what I do. I enjoy going into homes. I enjoy the people I work with. It brings me joy and happiness to know I am helping somebody."

Inadequate training and preparation was identified as a problem among study participants who fell into the "*It Works, But We Need More Support*" category. For example, a 59-year-old study participant who, while confident in her own skills, found training to be insufficient. She said:

> [We need] more training. I mean I'm familiar with strokes because of my family. I went through them with my family members. But not everyone is. And there was not mention of that, no training around that. But clients obviously go through that often. And then, the dementia should be required up front, because 50% of people are there or getting there.

Despite the recent increases in wages, compensation remained a key issue for the two study participants in the "*On My Way Out*" category. One

36-year-old study participant was actively looking for work outside the field of home care, in which she had worked for 16 years. While she had full time employment with health insurance, she described the benefits as not really being fair because, in order to keep the necessary 40 hours per week required to maintain health insurance, she needed to use her sick time when her clients' situations changed and she lost hours. She believed wages should be at least $15 per hour. She said:

> It makes me feel like I'm not valued, that I'm not worth enough. Because most people look at my financial situation and they says, "well why can't you get another job, or why can't you do this?" Does it matter to them that I already have three jobs and I'm working so hard? But when none of the those jobs pay a living wage, tell me one more time that I'm not working hard enough and I'm going to lose my mind.

The other study participant in this category left the field soon after our interview. She had worked in residential and home care for 34 years, but had never been able to move out of poverty as a single mother raising two children. She loved her clients and being a caregiver, but she was physically and emotionally exhausted from the work and her unsuccessful efforts to earn an adequate income.

Recommendations for Improving HCA Jobs

Both these studies underscored that HCAs find considerable fulfillment in their work, but are often forced to leave the field due to aspects of the job that could be improved. Offering increased compensation, access to health insurance, and more stability in hours are paramount for those workers who depend on their jobs for a living. The HCWRS revealed that older workers were less likely to leave their jobs in part as they often had other income (e.g., Social Security) supplementing their part-time home care work (Butler 2013). But for many workers, home care work is their only income, and some are relying on it to raise their children. Home care agencies are themselves struggling due to the low public investment in care for older adults and people with disabilities. Given that Medicaid funds a great portion of home care, increasing Medicaid reimbursement rates would allow home care agencies to pay their workers higher wages (Hess & Hegwisch 2019). Increasing federal and state minimum wages would also lead to higher wages for home care workers; this has been true in Maine where the minimum wage has increased more than four dollars over the past four years.

Guaranteeing health insurance, paid sick leave, and compensation for shifts cancelled at the last minute would contribute to the stability of the home care workforce. Lack of health insurance was one factor that significantly predicted termination in the HCWRS. Furthermore, many study participants noted the irony of working in the health field but not being able to take time off for their own health or that of their children when they were sick. First, they could not afford to miss work, as they had no paid time off, and second, they worried about their clients and whether there would be other HCAs to fill their shifts.

The national organization PHI (previously known as the Paraprofessional Healthcare Institute) has a mission to improve the jobs of direct care workers and to provide "quality care through quality jobs." A recent publication (Scales 2018) is directed towards employers of direct care workers, providing recommendations for recruiting and retaining a strong workforce. Their suggestions mirror those of the study participants in both the inquiries described in this chapter. They suggest providing employment supports such as on-site counselors and access to emergency loans. Peer mentorship is another recommendation, something that two study participants in the 2018 study wished were available to them as an advanced role; they each felt they had a lot to offer newly-hired workers. Peer mentorship programs both support newly hired workers' transition to their roles, and offer experienced workers a paid advancement opportunity (Scales 2018). Scales recommends offering other opportunities for advancement—with increased pay—such as creating the positions of senior aides and assistant trainers. Senior aides could provide problem-solving support to their peers and serve as a resource to interdisciplinary care teams;

assistant trainers would assist nurses in training by helping to facilitate skill-building and interactive sessions (Scales 2018).

Another recommendation put forward by Scales and PHI, effective supervision, would address some of the burnout issues described by HCAs in the two Maine studies described herein. They advocate a coaching style of supervision, which emphasizes building trust and respect, listening to a worker's perspective, engaging the worker in problem solving and developing action steps, while also monitoring performance (Scales 2018). Inviting the participation of employees in decision making and recognizing and rewarding them can also promote a work climate that promotes loyalty and ultimately retention.

We know the need for home care workers is going to continue to increase precipitously. We know that caring, hard-working individuals who do this work leave their jobs due to poor compensation or feeling undervalued by their employers, other health care professionals, and society. Solid recommendations for improving these jobs have been put forward and some have been implemented as pilot projects in different regions of the country. It is time for us to take national action and agree as a society that we need to invest in this workforce, so that the HCA job is appealing to potential new workers and sustaining for those already in the field. Any of us may require an HCA at some point in our lives; if we want to be sure there will be workers when we need them, we must support them in continuing to do the work they love.

REFERENCES

Butler, S. S. (2020). "Profiles of Women Who Help Us Age in Place." *Journal of Women & Aging*, *32*(1), 122-127.

Butler, S. S. (2013). "Older Women Doing Home Care: Exploitation or Ideal Job?" *Journal of Gerontological Social Work*, *56*(4), 299-317.

Butler, S. S., Wardamasky, S. & Brennan-Ing, M. (2012). "Older Women Taking Care of Older Women: The Rewards and Challenges of the Home Care Aide Job." *Journal of Women & Aging*, *24*(3), 1-22.

Butler, S. S., Simpson, N., Brennan, M. & Turner, W. (2010). "Why Do They Leave? Factors Associated with Job Termination Among Personal Assistance Workers in Home Care." *Journal of Gerontological Social Work*, *57*(8), 665-681.

Dawson, S. L. & Surpin, R. (2001). *Direct-Care Health Workers: The Unnecessary Crisis in Long-Term Care.* Bronx, NY: PHI.

Hess, C. & Hegewisch, A. (2019). *The Future of Care Work: Improving the Quality of America's Fastest Growing Jobs.* Washington, DC: Institute of Women's Policy Research.

Iezzoni, L. I., Gallopyn, N. N. & Scales, K. (2019). "Historical Mismatch Between Home-Based Care Policies and Laws Governing Home Care Workers." *Health Affairs*, *38*, 973-980.

Scales, K. (2019). *Envisioning the Future of Home Care: Trends and Opportunities in Workforce Policy and Practice.* Bronx, NY: PHI.

Scales, K. (2018). *Growing a Strong Direct Care Workforce: A Recruitment and Retention Guide for Employers.* Bronx, NY: PHI.

Seavey, D. & Marquand, A. (2011). *Caring in America: A Comprehensive Analysis of the Nation's Fastest Growing Jobs: Home Health and Personal Care Aides.* Bronx, NY: PHI.

Stacey, C. L. (2011). *The Caring Self: The Work Experiences of Home Care Adies*. Ithaca NY: Cornell University Press.

INDEX

A

acceptability, 2, 4, 13, 14, 21, 24, 25, 36, 41, 52, 56, 60
accreditation, xi, 88, 114, 124, 125, 127, 129
accreditation standards, 125
activities of daily living, v, vii, ix, 61, 62, 66, 71, 72, 75, 80, 83, 161, 196
aging, vii, ix, x, xii, 62, 64, 66, 77, 78, 79, 82, 86, 87, 92, 100, 103, 105, 106, 107, 109, 110, 113, 115, 129, 130, 131, 132, 133, 138, 154, 157, 158, 159, 160, 162, 163, 164, 165, 166, 170, 171, 176, 180, 193, 194, 197, 199, 207
assisted living, vii, ix, 2, 3, 6, 14, 15, 17, 23, 25, 28, 38, 41, 58, 59, 62, 72, 78, 139
assisted living homes, 139
assistive technologies, 62, 66, 73, 76, 77, 78, 84

B

basic education, 136, 145
burnout, xiii, 23, 28, 29, 32, 34, 35, 37, 38, 196, 199, 201, 202, 207

C

Canada, v, vii, xi, 52, 57, 81, 83, 107, 135, 137, 138, 139, 140, 141, 142, 144, 145, 147, 148, 149, 150, 152, 153, 154, 155
care assistants, xi, xiii, 38, 135, 137, 148, 178, 191
care providers, x, 3, 7, 30, 113, 137, 143
care quality, 2, 20, 23, 33, 37
care services, viii, xi, 1, 3, 5, 99, 127, 135, 137, 138, 139, 142, 150, 151, 164, 167
care workers, v, vii, xi, 32, 97, 135, 137, 138, 140, 144, 198, 203, 206, 207, 208
career advancement, xi, 135, 149
caring, 10, 28, 79, 91, 99, 105, 110, 115, 131, 136, 141, 163, 171, 192, 197, 207, 208
chronic pain, 170, 171, 172, 174, 175, 176, 179
community-based care system, 127
complaints, 24, 145, 146, 147
continuing training, xi, 135, 137

D

dependency ratio, 116
depression, 117, 119, 127, 170, 181, 187, 190, 193, 200
dominant infectious diseases, 116

E

elder care training, 142
elder carers, xi, 135, 137, 142, 145, 148
elderly, v, vii, ix, x, xii, 61, 62, 63, 64, 65, 66, 71, 72, 75, 76, 77, 78, 79, 80, 81, 82, 83, 86, 90, 97, 100, 105, 106, 109, 113, 114, 115, 116, 117, 118, 119, 120, 121, 122, 123, 124, 125, 126, 127, 128, 129, 130, 131, 136, 137, 138, 139, 140, 142, 144, 145, 147, 148, 149, 150, 152, 153, 154, 157, 159, 160, 164, 165, 167, 170, 172, 175, 176, 177, 180, 181, 189, 190, 191
elderly care workers, 136
elderly homes, x, 113, 114, 115, 117, 118, 119, 122, 124, 138, 140, 145, 149, 151
elderly homes in Lebanon, xi, 114, 117, 119
elderly homes medicine costs, 122
elderly people, vii, ix, xii, 61, 62, 63, 64, 65, 66, 71, 73, 75, 76, 77, 78, 81, 118, 136, 137, 138, 170, 175
elderly population, vii, 62, 64, 77, 116, 117, 118, 137
elderly wellbeing, 128, 136
end-of-service pension, 120
ethics, viii, 2, 3, 4, 5, 9, 11, 12, 14, 15, 16, 21, 26, 28, 29, 32, 33, 34, 35, 40, 41, 43, 44, 46, 50, 51, 52, 56, 60
extended care, 150

F

fall injuries, 145
family structure, 118, 123
fertility, 138
frail elderly, 108, 139, 151, 152
funding, 23, 87, 106, 120, 122, 151, 152, 172
furhter educational training, 136
further training, vii, xi, 135, 138, 141, 145, 147, 149

G

geriatric medical professionals, 119
geriatricians, 119
geriatrics, x, 103, 108, 110, 113, 120, 129, 148, 151, 169, 175, 176
geriatrics education, 151

H

happiness, vi, 76, 169, 204
health awareness, 128
health insurance, 116, 120, 122, 124, 198, 200, 204, 205, 206
health promotion, 128, 151
health workers, 120, 136, 144, 147, 148, 149, 150, 155
home care aides, viii, xiii, 195, 196, 198
home health, viii, xii, 177, 178, 180, 181, 182, 183, 188, 189, 190, 191, 192, 197
homes, xi, 114, 117, 119
human factors, viii, 2, 4, 5, 9, 10, 13, 14, 15, 16, 27, 36, 40, 45, 49, 59
human rights, 11, 47, 108, 128

I

in-kind resources, 122

intergenerational support, 127

L

Lebanese cultural pattern, 123
Lebanese older people, 115
Lebanon, v, vii, ix, x, 85, 86, 87, 88, 89, 93, 94, 95, 96, 97, 98, 99, 102, 103, 104, 105, 106, 108, 109, 113, 114, 115, 116, 118, 120, 121, 123, 124, 126, 127, 128, 129, 130, 131, 132, 133
licensed practical nurses (LPNs), 141, 144, 145
life expectancy, 114, 137
lifelong learning theory, xi, 136
long term care institutions, x, 113, 117
longevity, 138
long-term care settings, xi, 135, 141
lump-sum pension, 121

M

Maine, viii, xiii, 195, 196, 197, 199, 200, 203, 206, 207
malnutrition, 125, 126, 129, 130, 131, 133
medicare, vi, viii, xii, 150, 177, 178, 180, 181, 182, 183, 185, 186, 187, 188, 189, 190, 191, 192, 193, 197, 200
medication errors, 3, 20, 145, 146
minerals and vitamins deficiencies, 126

N

national social security fund, 120
non-communicable diseases (NCDs), 116, 117
non-formal social system, 123
nosocomial infections, 145, 151
NSWHN, 144, 152
nurses, xi, 38, 46, 95, 99, 100, 106, 108, 120, 135, 136, 137, 140, 141, 143, 144, 145, 146, 147, 148, 152, 153, 154, 178, 182, 187, 188, 190, 192, 207
nursing, 88, 89, 101
nursing home(s), v, vi, vii, ix, x, xi, xii, 42, 45, 82, 85, 86, 88, 89, 90, 91, 92, 93, 94, 95, 96, 97, 98, 99, 100, 101, 102, 104, 105, 106, 107, 108, 109, 110, 119, 126, 130, 131, 135, 137, 139, 142, 157, 158, 159, 160, 161, 162, 163, 164, 169, 170, 172
nursing staff, xi, 96, 97, 100, 102, 136, 139, 145, 147, 149
nutritional assessment, 126, 129, 133
nutritional status, xi, 114, 126, 129, 130, 132, 133
nutritional status of elderly, 125, 132

O

older adults, vi, viii, ix, xii, xiii, 3, 5, 8, 9, 11, 22, 29, 44, 52, 57, 59, 60, 61, 82, 86, 95, 96, 99, 106, 109, 110, 116, 117, 129, 131, 132, 138, 145, 146, 147, 149, 157, 158, 159, 160, 161, 162, 163, 164, 167, 169, 170, 171, 175, 176, 180, 193, 195, 206
older disabled people, 139
older women, 121, 123

P

pain, vi, viii, xii, 21, 92, 169, 170, 171, 172, 173, 174, 175, 176, 178, 186, 187
patient monitoring, 2, 10, 23, 37, 40
patient safety, viii, 1, 2, 3, 4, 7, 19, 23, 26, 27, 32, 33, 38, 42, 43, 44, 47, 55, 59, 60
patriarchal structure, 123
pension plan, 115, 121, 122, 127

population, vii, ix, x, xi, xii, xiii, 40, 41, 52, 57, 61, 62, 63, 64, 65, 78, 79, 80, 82, 85, 86, 87, 88, 98, 99, 101, 103, 113, 114, 115, 117, 118, 121, 122, 129, 131, 132, 133, 135, 138, 139, 140, 150, 152, 153, 155, 158, 159, 160, 162, 163, 164, 165, 166, 167, 171, 175, 176, 178, 180, 193, 195, 197, 200
population of Lebanon, 114
post basic education, 151
private and personal funding, 122

Q

quality, v, vii, viii, ix, x, xi, xii, 1, 3, 8, 23, 27, 29, 32, 37, 44, 46, 54, 58, 62, 63, 64, 66, 82, 85, 86, 87, 88, 89, 90, 91, 92, 93, 94, 95, 96, 97, 98, 99, 100, 101, 102, 103, 104, 105, 106, 107, 108, 109, 110, 114, 121, 124, 125, 126, 127, 128, 130, 131,135, 137, 140, 142, 143, 144, 145, 147, 148, 149, 150, 151, 153, 154, 155, 158, 162, 166, 175, 191, 192, 193, 206, 208
quality assurance control, 124
quality issues, 145, 151
quality of care, v, vii, viii, xi, 1, 3, 8, 37, 82, 104, 107, 128, 135, 137, 142, 143, 147, 148
quality of patient care, xi, 27, 136, 144

R

registered nurses (RNs), 141, 144, 145
registered psychiatric nurses (RPNs), 141, 145
residential care, ix, xi, 2, 5, 6, 7, 28, 46, 48, 55, 59, 85, 88, 92, 108, 109, 110, 135, 136, 137, 138, 139, 140, 141, 160, 163, 166, 167, 171, 175
retention, xiii, 34, 35, 196, 199, 203, 207, 208
risk of malnutrition, 126
role of the family, 115, 127

S

safety/risk assessment, 2, 40
skilled care workers, xi, 135, 137
smart cities, ix, 62, 64, 77, 78
smart homes, ix, 17, 62, 64, 66, 75, 76, 77, 78, 79, 83
social relationships, 119, 163
Social Security, 120
social security coverage, 122
social structure, 123
staffing, 146, 148
staffing level, 145, 146, 148
substance abuse, 178, 180, 181, 183, 185, 186, 187, 189, 190, 191
substance use, viii, xii, 177, 178, 179, 180, 181, 182, 183, 185, 186, 187, 189, 190, 191, 192, 194
surveillance, 8
surveillance technology, viii, 1, 2, 3, 8, 41

T

turnover, xiii, 92, 195, 198, 199, 200, 201

U

universal coverage, 150

V

video monitoring, viii, 2, 3, 13, 14, 15, 16, 20, 23, 27, 28, 31, 36, 37, 38, 40, 41, 42
vision systems, viii, 2, 3, 20, 37, 38, 41

W

wages, xiii, 120, 136, 196, 198, 200, 201, 203, 204, 206
welfare concept, 128
why this table or boxes?, 138